Vegan Cooking

Provides valuable nutritional advice for those on
a vegan diet as well as a complete range
of healthy and delicious recipes

Eva Batt

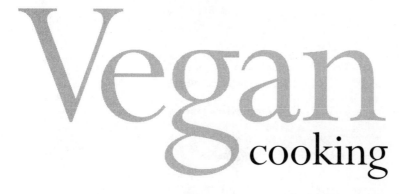

Vegan cooking

Recipes for Beginners

Thorsons

Thorsons
An Imprint of HarperCollins*Publishers*
77–85 Fulham Palace Road,
Hammersmith, London W6 8JB

The Thorsons website address is:
www.thorsons.com

and *Thorsons*
are trademarks of
HarperCollins*Publishers* Ltd

First published by Thorsons 1985
This edition published by Thorsons 2002

3 5 7 9 10 8 6 4 2

© Eva Batt 1985

A catalogue record of this book
is available from the British Library

ISBN 0 00 712997 1

Printed and bound in Great Britain by
Martins the Printers Ltd, Berwick upon Tweed

CONTENTS

ACKNOWLEDGEMENTS

In this book to all vegans, and the many vegans-to-be, I must first express my sincere appreciation of all the helpful advice and suggestions so willingly given by so many friends and colleagues.

In particular those doctors and nutritionists who have helped with the Introduction and friends and relatives who have contributed recipes and helped with tasting and testing.

It is my great hope that the many hours spent over a hot stove, testing, tasting and adjusting, will be rewarded by the knowledge that some of those thousands teetering on the brink of veganism will be encouraged, through the pages of this book, to take the plunge into the vegan world of *Eva Batt's Vegan Cookery*.

Whatever help this book may, or may not, be in introducing nourishing, flavoursome and economical dishes to budding vegans, I have learned a great deal in the process of compiling it.

FOREWORD

I am pleased to have the opportunity to write this passage as a commemoration to my mother, Eva Batt, and to the work she accomplished on behalf of veganism. In addition to this work, she had more than the usual share of domestic commitments, and her efficiency with which she despatched it all is a tribute to the improved energy and health that one has come to expect from the vegan diet. When I suggested that we needed a cookery book to aid people in their conversion, she took on the task at a time when her workload was already larger than herself (she was five foot nothing).

We hadn't expected the rush of sales that ensued when it was published, and quickly she had to have a reprinting to meet the demand. Those orders showed that people were already accepting that the vegan compass was pointing to the North; that thinking enquiring minds were recognizing that it works for the human good, better still, for the good of the whole. The continued demand for her book is evidence of how popular the vegan way of life has become.

Although the word 'Vegan' was contrived to separate vegans from lacto-vegetarians, the media spell it with a small 'v', affirming that it has become part of the language. I am thankful that veganism developed so well before mother died in 1989 (aged 81), when she saw for herself that her 30-year service was bearing the fruit that she and the Vegan Society had worked to produce. This book is a small part of her work, but in its reprinting she lives on for me, making it seem groundless to mourn her as I do. She would not wish me to still miss her, but that wish is ineffectual.

If you are just making the discovery that the human body was not designed to consume animal foodstuffs, then veganism is perhaps the greatest objective you could have to reach a more honest and meaningful future. In years to come, when you look back, in gratitude that you made the change, give a thought to the pioneers who had to do the groundwork, against opposition from all areas, to bring the truth to your attention. This book will make your transition a smooth and pleasant experience; the reason why it was written in the first place 20 years ago.

EVALAN WHITE

INTRODUCTION

These recipes are a selection of our 'first choice' meals and are planned for an economy budget. Economy need not mean dowdy meals, lack of flavour or low nutritional value.

If the suggested ingredient is temporararily priced high, out of season or scarce, it can easily be replaced with a similar one available at the time. In any case, fruit and vegetables in season are preferable.

If, conversely, a more glamorous dish is desired, it is a very simple matter to replace one vegetable with a more exotic one, aubergine, avocado, etc., or to add to it. Top a roast with slices of fried pineapple for instance.

Avocados are not exactly an economy food, but with their growing popularity they are becoming more widely distributed and cheaper. They are rich in essential fatty acids, contain a useful amount of protein and will convert a simple salad into a 'special' meal.

MINIMUM COOKING – MAXIMUM NUTRITION

This book is not intended primarily for the daily use of those following a food reform pattern. They will already appreciate the superior value of raw foods and plan their menus accordingly.

Nevertheless a well-prepared cooked meal can be a considerable help during the change-over period from a more orthodox diet, is more acceptable to non-vegetarian visitors, makes a pleasant change for anyone and is therefore of considerable value socially.

Furthermore, by preparing delicious dishes for those who have not yet adopted a food reform way of living we can demonstrate, in a practical and pleasant way, the wide variety of attractive and appetizing dishes which can be produced without the use of animal ingredients.

NUTS

Because of their unique properties, nuts can be eaten with almost anything. Ground, a little can be added to muesli, cakes or pastry mix, or stirred into soups and stews. Finely chopped they will improve any vegetable dish, or serve them whole or coarsely chopped with fruit salad, dried fruit or any dessert.

The above does not apply in the same degree to chestnuts or peanuts for the latter are not really nuts but legumes.

Nuts can also be baked or roasted. Almonds or cashews will quickly crisp and brown under the grill. Shake frequently to keep them turning.

Nuts are not an extravagance, they are a concentrated protein food, containing only about 10 per cent water compared with up to 50 per cent in flesh meats. Meat eaters often buy uneatable bone at high prices as well as a great deal of water. Furthermore, there is no waste in shelled nuts, no grisly bits, no objectionable odours and no putrefaction.

Both nuts and pulses are improved by being mixed with cereals, e.g., baked beans on toast. In such a combination the biological value of the protein is improved.

Nuts can usually be bought ready ground from a health food shop or good grocer. However, they will probably be fresher, and certainly cost less, if they can be ground at home. An electric blender or coffee grinder will do this very well.

COST OF HEALTH FOODS

Some people consider vegetarian protein foods such as nuts 'too expensive.' This is because they are accustomed to use them after a meal, as an 'extra.' When nuts are used in place of meat they will be found to be quite inexpensive by comparison.

Health foods, like anything else, can vary considerably in price.

Although ready-mixed Muesli and prepared tinned 'meats' may be useful on occasions, they are by no means necessary, and those prepared at home will not only cost less but the flavourings can be adjusted to suit the taste of the family. (We invariably find the pre-packed 'nut meats' are too highly spiced for our taste).

In general the less preparation bestowed on fresh, natural foods, the better.

Sweetcorn has a high nutritional value, being rich in vitamins A, B_1, B_2 and C. Ideally the kernels on the fresh cob should be in the creamy stage and suitable for eating raw. When not in season, the tinned or frozen kinds will add variety and nourishment to many dishes.

For the purpose of this book we include, under the heading 'Vegetables', all edible non-animal foods such as beans, seeds, herbs and fruits.

BEAN SPROUTS (AND SPROUTED GRAINS)

The sprouting of a variety of seeds and beans can be a very rewarding hobby, for these little fellows are among the most valuable and economical foods and readily available to everyone.

They can easily be grown anywhere, not even a window-box is required, whilst time, labour and cost are negligible.

Perhaps their greatest nutritional value lies in their high vitamin C content. The unsprouted grains, although a useful source of protein and B vitamins, contain very little vitamin C, yet after three to four days of growth this has increased by anything up to 600 per cent. The early mariners practised sprouting to ward off scurvy.

When seeds are sprouted the enzymic action separates the calcium and the phosphorus so that they can be more easily assimilated. This also happens to many other elements found in seeds. Iron is an example.

In most the peak of nutritonal concentration is reached by the third day, after which some of the nutriments are used to nourish the growing plants.

The starch in cereals is made more easily digestible by germination. If anything, the extra nutriment would increase the benefit (and calories) the consumer would derive.

Some of the quickest developers are the tiny pea-like mung beans or alfalfa (lucerne) grass seed. My family prefers the mung bean sprouts, and there is always a dish of them growing in the kitchen.

Special sprouting equipment can be bought, but is not necessary. All that is required is a small crock which can be easily washed — an earthenware soup bowl is ideal; an air permeable cover such as a piece of muslin — the seeds must have air; a few seconds of your time each day and a warmish place where they can germinate.

Glass is not the best container for, although it is easy to keep clean, the seeds need to be in the dark for most of the time.

Put about 2 tablespoonsful of the beans you have decided to sprout into your tray, dish, basin or whatever, cover with tepid water and leave to soak, covered, overnight (this quantity will fill a small basin when ready to eat).

In the morning rinse well in tepid water and strain off the surplus. Grains should be damp, but not lying in water. Do this twice more during the day and three times for each of the next two or three days. That is all.

Sprouts can be added to any food to its nutritional advantage: soups, savoury dishes and salads especially.

For practical purposes, sprouting confers these advantages:

1. Generation of vitamin C.
2. Breakdown of Phytic Acid (Phytin) and release of Calcium and Iron.
3. Increased digestibility.

Grains and beans suitable for sprouting can be bought from health food stores. Do not use seeds sold for sowing as these may be treated with mercurial compounds.

If not all the sprouts are required for immediate use they can be kept, covered, in the fridge for a day or two.

SUGAR

As with all sugars, cane sugar — that most guilty of all widely used vegetable foods — is harmless in its natural state, as it comes from the cane. Only after it has been refined, and lost all its minerals in the process, reduced to crystals and consumed in huge quantities, is it a menace to health.

The use of all refined sugars should be kept to an absolute minimum, and those who value their good health will train the palate to accept ever-reducing quantities.

White sugar contains only carbohydrates and nothing of nutritional value except calories.

Raw or Barbados sugar is a little better as it retains a small quantity of calcium and iron, but it cannot be considered a health food.

Our bodies require some unrefined sugar, and nature supplies adequate amounts in fruit complete with complementary vitamins and minerals. In many recipes dried fruit can entirely replace sugar, for example by adding raisins to muesli or porridge.

UNDERSTANDING PROTEIN REQUIREMENTS

I would like to be able to say that we all need 'X' quantity of protein daily and that this amount could be supplied by this or that food. Unfortunately, it is not quite that simple. First, our needs vary according to age, sex and occupation. The woman requires less than the man (as a rule), and the sedentary worker less than the coal miner or bricklayer. The experts tell us that the average adult should have 30-40 grams of protein a day, children and nursing mothers proportionately more.

Just as we can ensure adequate vitamins A and C by serving a variety of fresh green salads and fruit, our protein requirements would be met by including, during the day:

Some rice or other grain; one of the legumes such as haricot beans or lentils; some wholemeal bread; some wheat germ (added to bread, soup, muesli, etc.) and nuts — whole or in savoury, salad, or muesli dishes.

A selection of two or more items from these groups should be the aim. See the recipe pages for dishes in which these protein foods are featured.

Nuts are more beneficial when eaten raw as the amino-acid lysine is harmed when they are roasted.

EXAMPLE OF PLANNING

If breakfast included cereals and wheat germ and lunch consisted of a lentil savoury with wholemeal bread and a salad, the evening meal would, ideally, contain nuts in some form, either in a nut roast or just chopped and sprinkled on salad — green or fruit.

Although we are inclined to think only of certain foods in connection with proteins, we should remember that all food — with the exception of sugar, salt and possibly tea — contains some protein. In some cases only a trace, yet it will add to the daily intake. Of vegetables and fruits, avocados have the greatest amount, dried fruit and bananas a useful quantity, and passion fruit about twice as much as bananas.

Of nuts, chestnuts and coconuts, unlike all the others, are not a good source of protein — or fat for that matter, but are good food nevertheless.

The main thing to remember is to have as much variety as possible, and the recipes should help in this respect by introducing some new varieties of vegetarian foods, or new ways of serving old favourites.

'Peas, beans and lentils' is not just a catch phrase, but stands for nutritious food and a very economical source of protein in the diet. Collectively they are called the pulses.

It is best to serve two vegetable protein foods of different types at the same meal as this greatly increases the food value. For instance, one from the group of legumes and a grain such as rice or wheat.

Butter beans and haricots require longer cooking than red lentils. Rinse, soak overnight, and the following day cook in the same water, allowing up to two hours, although it does not always take as long as this. Red lentils will require only 20-30 minutes and need no pre-soaking.

SOYA

Soya flour is an excellent source of unsaturated fat, B vitamins, minerals and high quality protein. It enriches soups and sauces, and can be added to all savoury dishes and those calling for flour (bread, biscuits, cakes, etc.). Nutritionists recommend that soya beans be subjected to prolonged cooking under pressure, as used in the canning process. Ordinary kitchen equipment is usually unable to render them nutritionally suitable for regular use, and soya flour is normally the simplest way of using soya.

There is no danger from the tripsin inhibitor when using soya beans, as this is destroyed in the cooking. However, if using soya flour in an

13

uncooked recipe, such as soya cheese or marzipan sweets, make sure to get a brand which has been heat treated.

Food Combinations

Much has been written on the importance of selecting 'compatible foods' when planning meals, but the opinions of experts differ widely. Readers are strongly urged not to worry about it, this is more likely to disturb the digestion than a serving of apple pie.

The acid in a normal fruit dish is small compared with that in the stomach. The digestion works best if the acid in the stomach is neutralized by a protein dish (a main meal savoury) before it receives the starches (sweets), which is the form of the usual meal.

Foods are not usually incompatible in the stomach, even when they react visibly (e.g. lemon juice and vegetable milk). It is best to avoid such combinations that unbalance the supply of nutrients by over-loading the meal in carbohydrates.

There are some good combinations on which it might be wise to concentrate:

Vitamin A with fat . . . knob of fat on green vegetables.
Vitamin C with iron-containing foods . . . orange juice with stewed figs, fruit and nuts, etc.
Acid with calcium-containing foods . . . fruit fools, muesli, etc.
Pulse protein and cereal protein . . . beans on toast, nut meat.

It is good to take fat and vitamin D with calcium, as in bread and margarine. Flapjacks (made with oats and black treacle) are useful, cheap and pleasant sources of iron.

We all enjoy experimenting and creating our own 'family favourites' and it helps to know a little about which herbs blend most favourably with which vegetables; whether or not one is able to grow one's own — which is always preferable. Dill goes with cucumber of course, tomatoes are complemented by basil, caraway seeds for cabbage, parsley with carrots and, everyone's favourite, mint with new potatoes, peas and salads.

Carefully prepared meals, that one can offer with pride to guests unaccustomed to vegetable dishes, can be made even more attractive by the addition of a little — nutritious — decoration.

Garnishes

Grated Lemon and Orange Peel. Wash the fruit well in hot water first, if wax preservative has been used this will be seen to rise to the top of the water. Suitable for all fruit dishes and many desserts.

Chopped Parsley. Use on salads and any cooked dishes. Nutritious as well as decorative.

Finely Chopped Green Onions. For salads and savouries.

Fresh Mint. As above (adds vitamin C).

Slices of Mushroom, raw on salads or lightly fried on savoury dishes.

Fried Onion Rings. Shake in a bag of seasoned flour before frying for crispness.

Thin Rings cut from a fresh Green Pepper.

Tomato Slices uncooked or grilled.

Slices of fried Pineapple or Banana on hot savoury dishes.

Very thin strips of Red Pepper or **sliced ripe Olives** on salads or hot dishes.

Nutritional Values
Foods required for building and maintaining the body include:

> Calcium for the bones and teeth;
> Protein for the muscles; and
> Iron for the blood.

Protective foods are vitamins, fats and, to some extent, proteins. Food value charts vary a little because so many factors must be taken into account. Soil, weather, time of the year, country of origin, storage time (if any), drying or other processing, culture methods, etc. Nevertheless, it is very noticeable, when studying the resulting lists, that certain plant foods are outstanding in their nutritional value. For example:

> Almonds (iron, protein, calcium, thiamine, riboflavin, niacin).
> Brazils (calcium, protein).
> Cabbage (vitamin E, vitamin A, calcium).
> Peanuts (niacin, protein, calcium, riboflavin).
> Beans (calcium, protein, iron, vitamin A).
> Carrots (vitamin A).
> Dandelion Greens (vitamin A, vitamin C).
> Kale (vitamin A, vitamin C).
> Parsley, peas, red and green peppers, spinach, tomatoes and turnip greens are all valuable sources of vitamins A and C and some calcium.
> Figs (particularly black ones), dates, oranges, raisins and other dried fruits (calcium and iron).

Dried apricots (calcium, iron, vitamin A and vitamin C). Wholewheat flour and bread (protein, calcium, iron and carbohydrate).

VITAMINS, MINERALS AND OTHER NUTRIENTS

With two exceptions, vitamins and minerals are abundant in fruits and vegetables and we need have no concern regarding a possible deficiency in the diet. They also contain a variety of trace elements and valuable amounts of roughage (fibre).

The exceptions are vitamin B_{12} and vitamin D. Although a few people can manage without supplementing the diet, we recommend that some B_{12} fortified food is included in the diet. Some soya milks, yeast extracts and soya protein foods have added vitamin B_{12}. Although very little is needed by the body it is essential. One teaspoonful a day of a fortified yeast extract — used as a drink, a spread, added to savoury dishes or for flavouring soups and home-made soya cheese and nut butters — is adequate.

Because vitamin D is produced by the action of the sun on the oils in the skin (in any part of the body) exposure to this life-giving force should be taken whenever possible. Adults require little and are unlikely to lack vitamin D but growing children need more.

As the growing child requires more of some nutrients than the adult, nutritionists advise parents to ensure that children obtain adequate amounts of vitamins D, B_{12} and calcium.

Vitamin B_{12} tablets suitable for vegetarians are Cytacon 50 tablets, available at health food shops and chemists. Vitamin D drops are available from clinics. It is urged that parents take advice before giving these to children as too much can be dangerous.

MILK

Only breast milk contains perfectly balanced amino acids suitable for human babies. Cow's milk is not as well balanced — although ideal for calves — and, being mucus-forming, it is contra-indicated for those liable to colds, coughs and other respiratory complaints. However, milk of some kind is useful in cooking and drinks and the cholesterol-free vegetable milks are ideal, being useful sources of vitamin B_{12} as well as calcium and other nutrients.

CALCIUM

Molasses is a valuable source of calcium. Others include cress, cauliflower, dandelion leaves, swedes, turnips, cabbage, figs, dates, almonds, onions, parsley, carrots, kale, broccoli, sesame seeds, dried peas and beans and bread.

IRON

Parsley is very rich in iron so use it frequently, in soups, in roasts, on cooked vegetables and salads. Sadly it is often treated merely as a decoration and returned to the kitchen on the serving dish. Other inexpensive foods rich in this important mineral are lentils, sesame seeds, soya flour, black treacle, oatmeal, wheat flour, wholemeal bread, baked beans, cocoa, green peas, figs and apricots.

Sprouting is very useful for liberating nutrients and in generating vitamin C (e.g. in cereals and pulses). Also soaking the oats overnight for muesli helps absorption of the calcium and iron.

TEXTURED VEGETABLE PROTEIN (TVP)

There are now several brands available. Most come in flavoured and unflavoured varieties, in chunks and mince. Some of the flavoured kinds contain egg albumen or whey. It is advisable, therefore, to consult your copy of *The Vegetarian Handbook* or use only the unflavoured kinds. (If cooking for vegetarians, they will probably prefer not to have their food flavoured like meat in any case.)

A wide variety of savoury protein dishes can be made using tvp as a base, and tried old favourites given variety and added value by including this high protein food in pies, stews, puddings, goulash, curries and other dishes normally calling for meat.

Remember that this nutritious food is non-fattening (low in starch and fat), high in protein, economical, easily stored, requires very little cooking, and no waste (bone, skin, gristle or fat) is involved. Furthermore, there is no danger from added hormones or antibiotics, nor from bacterial food-poisoning.

When reconstituted with water, as the makers suggest, tvp contains 20-25 per cent protein, about the proportion in lean meat. Containing hardly any carbohydrate or fat, it is suitable for slimmers.

OILS AND FATS

Fats form an essential part of the diet, and the recommended vegan foods, including whole cereals, nuts, pulses, grains and the oils extracted from them, will supply all the types of fat required for health.

Home-made spreads and nut butters are very useful and, if necessary, the energy value of a diet can be improved by increasing the amount of vegetable oils, nuts or vegan margarine in this way. However, it should be remembered that excessive fat consumption encourages obesity as it has more than twice the number of calories per gram of either protein or carbohydrate.

For several reasons other than the avoidance of obesity, many people with certain heart and circulatory diseases are advised to reduce their intake of animal fats. In short, a near-vegan diet, although their practitioner may not call it that! In this respect vegans have an advantage over lacto-vegetarians, who often have high intakes of animal fats, i.e. milk, butter, cheese, cream and eggs.

For cooking, while a variety of oils high in polyunsaturates is best, a proportion of *Nutter* or *Suenut*, as used in some of the recipes in this book to produce the best results in texture, is permissible.

For convenience, manufacturers are being urged to introduce soft spreads without the whey or milk solids — commonly used for flavouring — and hopefully some of these will be available before long.

'OUR DAILY BREAD'

Make it at home from 100 per cent wholemeal flour (not just brown), for the flour in the commercially made white loaf will have been denuded of twenty nutrients in the process of refining and bleaching. The law requires that four of these must be returned to the flour, leaving us with a nutritionally unbalanced food even before the baker adds the 'improvers', 'mould inhibitors', 'emulsifiers', 'maturing agents', 'conditioners', 'stabilizers', 'extenders', 'softeners', chalk, etc. Not to mention the lard which is commonly used in the baking.

'I WOULD BE A VEGETARIAN IF I COULD AFFORD IT'

'If meat gets any more expensive we shall all have to become vegetarians' is a joking remark frequently heard in these days of rising prices. It demonstrates our basic realization that a diet which includes flesh food is more costly than others, yet few people are aware just how wasteful, in labour, money and actual food, is the process of rearing food animals for human consumption.

But for the subsidies which support the economy this would be far more apparent to the consumer, but whether we pay the butcher the real price of his wares or pay part of the cost in taxes, the high cost of production remains the same.

It is the wastage of food which should be our chief concern, for cattle will consume five to ten times as much food (grass and grain) as they eventually provide in the form of meat. This is real waste in a world where so many are sadly undernourished.

If we have no thought for the animals bred and slaughtered by the million, quite unnecessarily, to satisfy the western palate, the knowledge that hungry children are being even further deprived by these practices will surely be enough to make us all think again about adopting a more humane, and healthy, diet.

CATERING FOR ONE ON A SLIM BUDGET

This can be a problem for a person on a mixed diet for it is not possible to buy half a lamb chop, and a request for one joint from an ox tail would probably raise a lot of eyebrows. But the vegetarian has no need to shop daily for very small pieces of fish or whatever. The vegetable protein foods (see page 20) including the soya-based meat-like tvp, have a very good shelf life and can be kept until required, thus saving shopping time for the busy person. What is perhaps more important is that recipe quantities can be easily reduced (or expanded when necessary) whereas it would be difficult to 'take a quarter of an egg'!

SLIMMING 'DIETS'

The vegetarian diet, as such, does not claim to be a slimming programme, containing as it does both high and low calorie foods. Nevertheless, the number of overweight vegetarians seems to be very small indeed. That is probably because, when a person becomes sufficiently interested in food to adopt this way of life, he or she will also appreciate the importance of food reform in general and will increase their consumption of fresh vegetables while indulging less frequently in puddings, pies and sweets.

Anyone counting calories will concentrate mainly on those protein foods with rather less fat content: defatted soya flour, textured soya protein, baked beans, peanuts, although not exclusively of course. For slimmers also, a variety of foods is essential and plenty of salads should be included in the diet.

All green vegetables, with the exception of green peas, are among the very low calorie foods and all fruits (except bananas) can also be included in this group. Mushrooms are more calorie-shy than any other food, so would make a useful addition to the meal for those wishing to lose weight.

Essential Nutrients from Vegetable Sources

Proteins

For growth and the repair of body tissues, and for energy. Their physical properties may be changed by cooking and food preparation generally.

Found in appreciable amounts in nuts, yeast, grains, seeds, legumes, wheatgerm, flour and bread.

Fats

For energy, heat and to assist in the absorption of fat soluble vitamins and calcium.

Found in vegetable oils, nuts and nut creams, cooking fats, nut butters and margarine, and vegan white fats, available from grocers.

Essential Fatty Acids
(e.g. linolenic and arachidonic acids)

These limit the formation of excess cholesterol in the blood. They are sources of the prostaglandins which regulate processes in the smooth muscles.

Found almost exclusively in vegetable oils: peanuts, sesame, sunflower and safflower seeds and the derived oils and fats.

Note: The essential fatty acids (EFA, once called vitamin F) are polyunsaturated. Other unsaturated fats occur mainly in vegetable oils. Although these are not essential, their consumption is to be preferred over that of saturated fats, in order to prevent high levels of cholesterol in the blood and coronary and circulatory troubles. Vegetable oils are therefore to be preferred to any animal fats. The oils from coconuts and olives are the only vegetable oils with a high content of saturated components.

Carbohydrates

For energy. Excess may cause overweight.

In all cereals including bread and flour products, dried fruits, dried peas and beans, bananas, sugar, potatoes and others.

Protein, fat and carbohydrate combine to form calories — which supply heat and energy.

IRON

For proper formation of red blood cells and regulation of body processes.

Whole grain cereals, black treacle, raisins, nuts, sesame seeds, soya flour, pulses, cocoa, curry powder.

CALCIUM

For the development and growth of bones and teeth, normal clotting of blood and functioning of muscles.

In spinach, molasses, sesame seeds, parsley, almonds, soya flour, Brazils and other nuts and 'greens'.

TRACE ELEMENTS

Essential accessories to vital processes and to action of other nutrients.

In a wide range of foods, especially unrefined.

VITAMIN A
(or Carotenes)

For growth in children, it plays a part in the way the eyes receive light, protects moist surface tissues (bronchial tubes, etc.).

Found in carrots, watercress, dried apricots, prunes, tomatoes, cabbage, green peas, all green vegetables and margarine.

VITAMIN B_1
(Thiamine)

For growth, appetite, digestion, and the nervous system.

In bread and wheat products, pulses generally, yeast (brewer's is best), Brazils and peanuts (uncooked), wheat germ.

VITAMIN B_2
(Riboflavin)

For vitality, healthy skin, growth and good sight.

In yeast, lentils, rye, mushrooms, parsley, broccoli tops, and green vegetables generally.

NICOTINAMIDE

For healthy digestion, good skin condition, and growth.

In soya, peanuts, flour and bread, yeast, rice, pulses generally and beer.

Folic Acid

Prevents certain kinds of anaemia, assists growth.

In all green vegetables, yeast extracts.

Vitamin B$_{12}$

For growth, nerve cells and the prevention of certain kinds of anaemia.

In fortified foods such as *Plamil*, vegetable milks, yeast extracts and several kinds of textured vegetable protein.

Vitamin C

For healing wounds, prevention of scurvy, maintaining stamina, strong blood vessels, resistance to infection.

Citrus fruits, tomatoes, soft fruits, red and green peppers, leafy greens, potatoes.

Vitamin D

Building bones and teeth. Growth.

From sunshine, fortified vegetable milks and all margarines and soft spreads.

Vitamin E

Growth, muscle tissues, normal reproduction. Possibly retards ageing.

Wheat germ, whole grain cereals, green leafy vegetables.

Vitamin K

Regulates clotting of blood.

In green leafy vegetables.

Fibre

Keeps vascular system in good tone, i.e. prevents troubles in the intestines, veins and arteries.

In unrefined foods, especially cereals (e.g. bran).

These are just a few examples for use as a general guide if required when planning menus.

The above notes are, of necessity, brief. A fuller picture with helpful charts, is contained in the booklet *Vegan Nutrition* by T.A.B. Sanders, B.Sc. Nutrition, Ph.D., and the late F.R. Ellis, M.D., F.R.C. Path. Published by The Vegan Society, 7 Battle Road, St Leonards-on-Sea, East Sussex, TN37 7AA.

KITCHEN HINTS

● No special cooking utensils are required in the vegan kitchen, but, if funds allow, a juicer is extremely useful. It enables the owner to extract the nutrients from the parts of vegetables and fruit which, mostly because of an unattractive appearance, would be discarded, i.e. windfalls, outside leaves of celery, cabbage, lettuce, etc. Apart from using the juice as a refreshing drink, diluted it makes an excellent stock for soup, particularly a fresh, cold soup (Gazpacho).

● Another useful aid is an electric blender (liquidizer). It will chop nuts, make breadcrumbs or purée vegetables. Both these aids save time and work but are not essential.

● Breakfast Muesli can be prepared overnight except for the addition of fresh fruit, which should be added to the cereals and nuts just before serving.

● The good cook will not, of course, throw away any vegetable water after cooking, but use it in other dishes. In this way at least the minerals released into the water during cooking are not wasted.

● A baked, unsweetened apple will add piquancy to any savoury dish, a sliced grilled tomato will give colour and flavour to one which seems to lack it, and just any dish will look more attractive and taste even more delicious if topped with a slice of fried pineapple.

● Don't be afraid to mix fruit and vegetables. Try diced raw apple with any spiced dish such as curry and thin slices of orange will complement hot dishes as well as salads. Use peaches or grapes in this way when in season.

● A little cider vinegar added to the washing water will help remove pesticides from commercially grown vegetables.

● When making cakes a little soya flour helps to emulsify the fat.

● Tahini is rich in calcium and, weight for weight, contains more than milk solids.

● Celebration cakes. Replace egg whites with agar agar dissolved in water for royal icing.

● Boiling will remove any sulphur dioxide from dried fruit. Fruit with a glossy appearance has most likely been treated with liquid paraffin but currants and muscatels are not normally so treated.

● A little salt added to the water when cooking pasta or rice will make water boil more vigorously and help to stop the food sticking. Do not, however, add salt while cooking beans as they will take longer to soften if you do. But salt can, of course, always be omitted for persons on a low-salt or salt-free diet.

- For beans an overnight soak may be sufficient, but to ensure giving enough time for this , allow 24 hours. Split peas and lentils need not be soaked. For soups, stews and casseroles just wash and add to the other ingredients to cook. If to be cooked alone, allow 4 oz (115g) lentils to about 1 pint (570ml) water (some take a little more). Simmer for 20 minutes or until tender and water is all absorbed. Here again the time will vary a little, it is helpful therefore if these high protein foods are prepared in advance of the rest of the meal. Do not leave the lentils unattended for long during cooking though, as they may froth 'up and over'. Stir frequently to avoid sticking. A little oil in the water will minimize this.

FRYING

Although frying is not the best way to prepare food, we are going to use this method occasionally unless it is banned for health reasons — and a few suggestions on frying may be useful.

Always use oil. Deep frying is best whenever possible. For this use a heavy pan and fill only one third with oil. Except for potatoes, coat the food in batter first to retain nutrients. Have oil at correct temperature (360°F/180°C) which is reached when a chip, when placed gently in the pan, rises almost immediately. Do not wait for oil to smoke. Lower heat before lowering food. Well blot chips to dry and put no more than will cover the bottom of the basket at one time. More food than this will lower the temperature too suddenly. Fry for approximately 6 minutes then, for a crisp, brown finish, raise the heat a little for another 4-5 minutes.

For shallow frying pancakes and fritters use a very little oil in a heavy pan on medium heat. This will be ready for frying in one minute. Do not raise the heat.

SAUTÉ POTATOES

Use 5-6 tablespoons oil on a medium heat. Ready for frying in about 4 minutes (or when a 1 inch/2cm cube of bread takes 15 seconds to turn golden brown on one side).

If partially cooked the potatoes should be ready in 3-4 minutes. If raw, reduce heat to low and cook for 9-10 minutes.

FATS

When replacing margarine with oil in pastry or cake recipes it should be remembered that approximately 25 per cent less will be required, i.e. 3 fl oz (90 ml) of oil is the equivalent of 4 oz (115g) of margarine.

Make your own nut butters. Put chopped nuts in blender at high speed. Gradually add a little oil. The amount needed will vary according to the nuts used.

DRIED FRUIT

Sun-Maid seedless raisins are recommended as they are not treated with mineral oil and are naturally sun-dried. If any dried fruit appears unusually shiny, the oil coating can be removed by washing in warm water, when it will be seen to float to the surface.

The dried fruits: dates, prunes, raisins, etc., are a good source of immediate energy and do not have the lowering after-effects of refined cane sugar.

LABELLING

It is advisable to read carefully the labels on packed foods, as in many cases it is not clear whether the named ingredients are of animal or vegetable origin. Happily the vague term 'edible fats' is no longer accepted on lists of ingredients in packed foods, but often the present 'E' coding system is no more helpful. For instance lecithin has the code number E322 regardless of whether it is derived from soya beans or eggs. Similarly, where vitamin D is added to a food the manufacturer should be asked to state if it is vitamin D_2 (vegan) or D_3, which is not! In the interest of clearer labelling it is recommended that individuals approach the manufacturer concerned, requesting more explicit information on vague statements.

Ascorbic Acid (vitamin C) — Occurs naturally in many fruits and green vegetables, also potatoes, expecially new potatoes. Also produced synthetically from vegetable or mineral sources, not animal.

Collagen — An insoluble protein in bones, tendons, skin and connective tissue of animals. Converted to bone gelatin by heat.

Farina — Starch, generally in the form of flour. Derived mostly from potatoes.

Gelatin (See Collagen) — A tough gelling agent used for encapsulated fruit flavourings, vitamin supplements, ice cream and desserts such as mousse.

Glucose Glycerol — A sweet liquid obtained by decomposition of fats and distillation. Unlikely to be of vegetable origin.

Glycerol Monostearate — Emulsifying agent obtained by partial decomposition of fats or by combination of glycerol and stearic acid. Not necessarily vegetable, but used largely in the manufacture of commercial ice cream, desserts, biscuits, bread and margarine.

Hydrolized Vegetable Protein — Derived largely from cereals, for flavouring soups, etc.

Lactose — Milk sugar used widely in baby foods and confectionery.

Lecithin — An emulsifier and stabilizer. It occurs in eggs and for use as an additive in other foods, is obtained from soya beans, peanuts and corn. The addition of a little soya flour in savouries, soups, bread, etc., will ensure that adequate lecithin is included in the diet.

Monosodium Glutamate — One of the naturally occurring amino acids of vegetable origin. Used to bring out meaty flavours. As with other sodium additives, its overuse could upset the body's sodium/potassium balance. A certain — harmless — amount would be naturally present, not added, in yeast extracts and similar flavourings.

Pectin — A light gelling agent found in fruits and plants. Used as a basis for vegetable jelly and in preserves and for clarifying fruit juices and wines.

Sodium Alginate — A seaweed extract used to thicken foods and as an emulsifier.

Sodium Caseinate — Prepared from milk and used as an emulsifier and stabilizer.

Sulphur Dioxide — A gas used as a preservative for fruits and vegetables. Stabilizes vitamin C, but destroys vitamin B_1.

Sodium Sulphate and **Sodium Metabisulphate** — These are solid forms (e.g. Camden tablets).

Calcium Chloride — Usually derived from calcium carbonate by reaction with hydrochloric acid. A crisping agent.

Polysorbates — Emulsifiers and stabilizers containing polyoxyethylene sorbitan and fatty acids. Used in cake mixes, toppings and confectionery.

'Permitted' dyes, flavourings, anti-scaling agents, etc., are those which are 'innocent because they have not yet been proven guilty'. Which additives are 'permitted' depends on the country in which you happen to be, for the experts are divided as to which of the 2,000 odd comparatively new food additives can be consumed safely — and which cannot.

MUESLIS

Breakfast muesli can be prepared overnight except for the addition of fresh fruit and nuts. Fruit should be stirred into the mixture just before serving and the nuts sprinkled on top. Mix or vary the kind of nuts used remembering that almonds have the highest protein content and that hazel nuts blend best with fruit. If the family dislike the skins they can be easily rubbed off the latter if the nuts are slightly roasted first. To remove almond skins, cover with boiling water for a few minutes and twist off the skins whilst still wet. Nuts do not need to be skinned, we always leave them on unless they are used for decoration on cakes, etc.

Pears or apples should be quickly and coarsely grated and stirred into the muesli cereals straight away to prevent discolouration. Flavour variety can be gained by the addition of freshly grated orange or lemon peel (wash fruit in hot water first) or rosehip or blackcurrant syrup. The good cook supplies continuous variety, even with breakfast muesli. Apricots are an excellent food. If rather dry they can be soaked for a few hours with a little lemon rind.

For added nutrition — and as an aid to natural elimination — add a little bran (untreated wheat bran and the germ naturally present) to soups, breakfast cereals, savouries, bread, cakes, biscuits, etc. A selection of muesli bases can be bought at health shops.

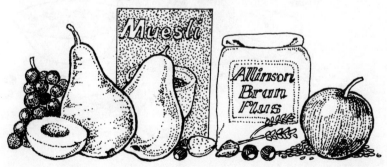

Beauty Breakfast

3 oz (85g) apricots, previously soaked if
necessary
1 tablespoon muesli base
3 tablespoons vegetable milk
1 teaspoon lemon juice
2 teaspoons Barbados sugar (optional)
1 banana
1 tablespoon almonds, halved or grated

1. Mince, liquidize or well chop apricots.
Add cereal base and mix well.

2. Add milk, juice and sugar. Stir again.

3. Add sliced banana and lastly, add nuts but
do not stir in.

Note: For diabetics half the recipe quantity
of a fruit sugar can be used in place of cane
sugar. This does not utilize insulin as does
cane sugar.

Apple Muesli

1 large or 2 small apples
1 tablespoon almond or cashew cream
diluted in 3 tablespoons water
1 tablespoon raw oatmeal for each
person, pre-soaked
1 tablespoon lemon juice
2 teaspoons Barbados sugar (or 1 teaspoon
fruit sugar for diabetics)
1 tablespoon chopped nuts

1. Wash and dry apples.

2. Put nut cream into bowl and add water
slowly while stirring.

3. When emulsified, add cereals.

4. Add lemon juice and sugar, stir.

5. Roughly grate apples and add, stirring
in immediately. Sprinkle on nuts and
serve.

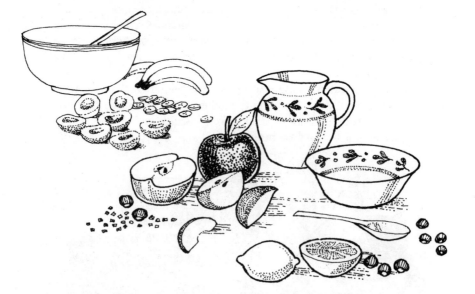

Muesli with Dried Fruit
(Prepared Overnight)

2 oz (55g) dried fruits which have been previously washed (apricots, prunes, raisins, apple rings, etc.)
A little grated orange or lemon peel
1 tablespoon lemon juice
2 teaspoons Barbados sugar
1 tablespoon muesli base or whole rolled oats

1. Chop, liquidize or mince soaked fruit.

2. Add peel, lemon juice and sugar and stir into cereals. Add water to cover.

3. In the morning serve with a few chopped nuts sprinkled over.

Note: Vegetable milk or blackcurrant syrup can be added at table.

Fresh Fruit Muesli
(Rich in vitamin C)

4-5 oz (115-140g) fresh fruit (apples, strawberries, raspberries, black or red currants, peaches, apricots, bananas, oranges)
2 teaspoons Barbados sugar
2 tablespoons vegetable milk (or water)
1 tablespoon muesli base (pre-soaked for preference)
1 tablespoon grated hazel nuts

1. Wash fruit and trim as necessary. Chop small, slice or mash with wooden spoon according to fruit being used.

2. Mix in the sugar and the milk. Add the cereal base and mix thoroughly.

3. Sprinkle nuts over finished dish and serve immediately. This dish is strongly recommended for the sedentary worker and those prone to skin troubles.

Well wash any kind of dried fruit and soak overnight in orange or lemon juice. Delicious with breakfast muesli — or any other time.

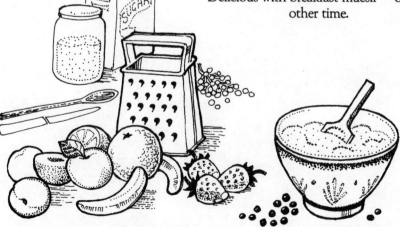

Soups and Small Savouries

'Stock' is the water in which vegetables have been cooked, either for the table or, in the case of coarse outside leaves, to be discarded after being strained from the stock — in which will remain much of their valuable content and flavour.

A few sample soups are given here but many other combinations will suggest themselves. Ring the changes with vegetables, almost anything to hand can go in. Just scrub and shred, the finer they are grated the sooner the soup will be ready for the table, but any vegetable soup should not take more than 30 minutes to prepare.

As with all non-animal foods, soups are spoiled by over-cooking.

Strain for clear soup: sieve or liquidize and add cashew nut cream or peanut butter and 2 teaspoons of barley flour or fine oatmeal for cream or thick soups.

If grated or finely chopped vegetables have been used these can be left in and the soup thickened with soya flour to make, with wholemeal bread, a quick and satisfying meal.

Clear or cream soups can be made more attractive with a simple garnish. Tiny shreds of celery, chopped chives or mint, parsley or watercress leaves floated on the surface, or thin slivers of red or green peppers are ideal.

At table, serve with wheatgerm, sea salt, sprouted grains, bran or kelp powder, any of which can be added to taste.

BASIC SOUP

2 tablespoons vegetable oil
1 onion, scrubbed and chopped
(about 6 oz/170g)
Several stalks of celery, chopped (use the
less attractive outside stems for this
purpose)
1½ pints (850ml) vegetable stock or water
2 potatoes, scrubbed and sliced
(about ½ lb (225g)
2 bay leaves
1 teaspoon sea salt
2 good tablespoons bean sprouts

1. Heat oil in pan and cook the onion and
celery for 10 minutes, shaking frequently.

2. Add stock, potatoes, bay leaves and
salt. Bring to the boil and simmer until
just cooked; never over-cook.

3. Remove bay leaves, strain soup and rub
through sieve or liquidize in blender for a
few seconds. Reheat adding sprouts and
serve as soon as possible.

ONION AND LENTIL SOUP

½ lb (225g) onions
2 oz (55g) vegetable oil
1 medium sized carrot
2 pints (1.1 litre) vegetable stock
½ lb (225g) lentils
Yeast extract
Seasoning

1. Peel the onions, cut into small pieces
and cook in the oil until soft, together
with the carrot cut small.

2. Add the vegetable stock and lentils and
cook until they are soft.

3. Rub through a sieve and return to the
pan.

4. Add yeast extract and seasoning to
taste.

GAZPACHO

1 small green pepper
1 medium onion
2 tablespoons vegetable oil
½ pint (285ml) tomato purée (skin
tomatoes and put through blender)
1 clove garlic, crushed (optional)
A small quantity of any other vegetables
to hand, such as courgettes or okra
5 oz (140g) cucumber
A few slivers of lemon peel and juice to
taste
Seasoning
A few watercress leaves

1. Wash pepper, remove seeds and cut into
small pieces.

2. Skin, chop and sauté onion in the oil.
(About 5 minutes).

3. Add the peppers to the onion and the
skinned, chopped tomatoes. Cook for a
further 5 minutes.

4. Add other ingredients, except
cucumber and lemon juice, and simmer
for 15-20 minutes.

5. Remove lemon rind, add juice and
seasoning to taste. Chill, then just before
serving float the watercress leaves on top.

Note: Serve with the cucumber, finely
diced, in a separate dish. Guests will be
pleased to add this to their liking.

Leek and Lentil Soup

Leeks (about 6 oz (170g) when trimmed)
3 teaspoons vegetable oil
1 pint (570ml) stock or water
4 oz (115g) red lentils
Sea salt
Bouquet garni

1. Cook leeks in oil gently in heavy covered pan for 10 minutes, stirring frequently.

2. Add 1 pint stock or water, lentils, 1 teaspoon sea salt and a bouquet garni (from health food shops). Simmer for 20-30 minutes.

3. When lentils are soft remove herbs and liquidize or press through sieve. Add 1 teaspoon yeast extract for extra flavour if desired.

Parsnip Soup

2 leeks
1 parsnip (about 6 oz)
2 tablespoons vegetable oil
1½ pints (850 ml) stock
1 large potato (about ½ lb /225g)
Sea salt

1. Wash and trim leeks and parsnip, cut fairly small and sauté in the oil for 5 minutes or so.

2. Add stock, scrubbed, sliced potato and salt. Simmer until tender — do not over-cook.

3. Press through sieve, reheat and just before serving, add watercress leaves and any of the following: bean sprouts, wheat-germ or soaked whole wheat.

Potato and Onion Soup

½ lb (225g) onions, chopped small
1 head celery, chopped
2 tablespoons vegetable oil
1½ pints (850ml) stock
½ lb (225g) potatoes
2 bay leaves (large ones)
Celery salt (optional)

1. Cook onions and celery in oil for 10-15 minutes with lid on pan.

2. Add stock, potatoes, scrubbed and cut up, and bay leaves. Simmer for 20-30 minutes.

3. Sieve, add celery salt, and reheat. Garnish with chopped chives or parsley if liked.

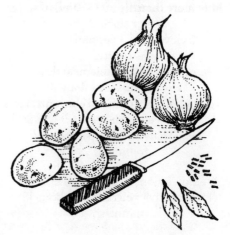

PARSNIP CREAM SOUP

1 lb (455g) parsnips
1 large onion
1 oz (30g) vegan margarine or oil
2 pints (1.1 litres) stock
Bay leaf
Sea salt
2 good teaspoons nut cream
1 teaspoon yeast extract

1. Scrub and slice parsnips and onions. Cook gently in margarine or oil for 10 minutes.

2. Add stock, bay leaf and salt. Simmer until cooked, add nut cream and yeast extract. Stir until dissolved.

3. Rub through sieve. Reheat and garnish with chopped chives or watercress leaves.

CREAM OF ONION SOUP

1 lb (455g) onions
A little more than 1 pint (570ml) of water or stock
2 cloves and 3 peppercorns
Seasoning
½ oz (15g) 81% wholemeal flour
2 teaspoons soya flour
¼ pint (140ml) undiluted concentrated vegetable milk
A good handful chopped parsley (optional)

1. Chop onions. Cook in water with cloves and peppercorns for about 15 minutes.

2. Remove spices and sieve. Add seasoning.

3. Cream flours with a little cold water and blend, stirring, with the onion liquid. Bring gently to the boil and simmer for a few minutes.

4. Add milk and reheat without boiling. Add chopped parsley just before serving.

BARLEY CREAM SOUP

1 medium onion
3 sticks celery
1 carrot
2 tablespoons vegetable oil
2 pints (1.1 litres) stock or water
2 oz (55g) pot barley
Seasoning
Small teaspoon yeast extract

1. Peel and chop the onion, cut the celery and carrot into small pieces and fry with the onion in the oil for about 10 minutes.

2. Add the stock and barley and simmer until the barley is soft — about 2½ hours.

3. Sieve or liquidize and return to the pan, add seasoning, yeast extract and decorate with chopped parsley or watercress leaves.

Salads and
Salad Dressings

There would appear to be little need in a cookery book for a chapter on raw salads, but too often I find, particularly in the average restaurant, that this dish is confined almost exclusively to lettuce, tomato and cucumber. This is a pity when there is such a wide variety of suitable ingredients. I have therefore included a few suggestions which will not only add interest to the salad meal, but provide an ample supply of all the vitamins and minerals.

If not included in the recipe, some kind of protein food should be added. It could be just grated nuts, a lentil rissole or a soya savoury.

Jacket potatoes make a good accompaniment to salads, or home-made bread with margarine and a savoury pâté, or yeast extract are excellent.

First a few reminders of some of the many fruits and vegetables suitable for inclusion in what is probably the most important meal of the day — the raw salad.

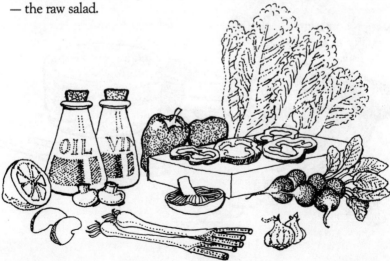

A Few Salad Ingredients

Shred	Slice	Chop	Grate
Broccoli (young leaves)	*Avocado	Apple	Beetroot (raw)
Brussel sprouts	Batavia	*Celery	Brussel sprouts
Cabbage — red or green	Banana	*Chestnuts	Carrots (raw)
Cauliflower heads	Beetroot (cooked)	Chives	Celeriac (raw)
Dandelion (young leaves)	Carrots (cooked)	*Dates	Garlic (or crush)
*Endive	Chicory	Herbs (fresh)	Onion
Leeks	Cucumber	Jerusalem artichokes	
*Lettuce	Fennel	*Nasturtium leaves	
*Okra	Melon	Mooli	
Peppers (red and green)	Orange	*Nuts of all kinds	
*Runner beans (young)	Pears	Pineapple	
*Watercress	Pineapple	*Radishes	
	*Tomatoes	Salsify	
	Potatoes (cooked)	*Spring Onions	

*These items may be left whole. The minimum of chopping or cutting helps to preserve vitamins. Many can be chopped, sliced, shredded or grated.

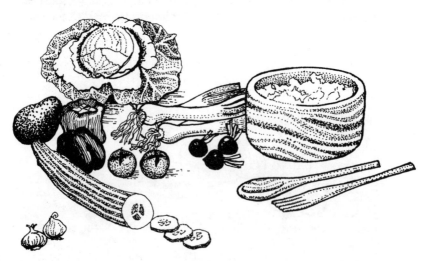

36

Pear, Date and Nut Salad

3 ripe dessert pears
1 small crisp lettuce
4 oz (115g) chopped dates
2 oz (55g) chopped walnuts
Chopped parsley
Oil and lemon dressing

1. Peel and halve the pears, remove the cores and scoop out a little pulp to leave a hollow for filling. (The pulp can be mixed into the filling).

2. Shred finely a few lettuce leaves and mix with the dates, nuts, parsley and pulp, then add oil and lemon to taste.

3. Put the halved pears on a bed of lettuce leaves and pile the mixture onto each of them. Sprinkle the halved pears with lemon juice to prevent discoloration while they are waiting for filling.

Banana, Raisin and Carrot Salad

2 or 3 bananas
1 oz (30g) seedless raisins
1 oz (30g) almonds
1 carrot (approx. 3oz/85g)
mayonnaise
Chopped parsley

1. Slice the bananas thinly and mix in the washed raisins, coarsely chopped nuts, and finely grated carrot.

2. Pile in the salad bowl, add mayonnaise to taste, and sprinkle lavishly with parsley.

Apricot Salad

4 oz (115g) dried apricots
1 small to medium cauliflower
3 medium tomatoes
4 oz (115g) cooked peas
1-2 oz (30-55g) choppd walnuts
2 tablespoons vegetable oil
1 tablespoon lime juice (or lemon juice)
1 teaspoon raw cane sugar

1. Wash and blot dry the apricots and cut into slices. Break cauliflower into florettes. Cut tomatoes into wedges.

2. Mix the oil, lime juice and sugar to make the dressing. Shake well.

3. Toss the ingredients in dressing.

4. Serve tossed ingredients on a bed of endive (or lettuce). Decorate with small sprigs of watercress.

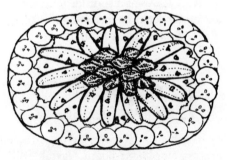

Banana Salad

Cover the bottom of a flat dish with watercress or lettuce. Cut some bananas in halves and then in four lengthways. Arrange these on the lettuce radiating from the centre. Pile stoned dates in the centre and, around the outside edge, overlap thin slices of cucumber. Sprinkle with chopped nuts. Serve with mayonnaise.

Orange Waldorf Salad

1 large orange
½ red dessert apple
Celery heart
Few seedless raisins
1 teaspoon each of orange and lemon juice
1 teaspoon vegetable oil
1 teaspoon soft brown sugar
Lettuce

1. Peel and dice the orange, dice the apple, and mix both with the chopped celery and raisins.

2. Make the dressing from the orange and lemon juice, oil and sugar.

3. Arrange the fruit mixture on a bed of lettuce leaves and sprinkle with the dressing, or serve in the orange shell with a lettuce surround.

Quick and Easy Coleslaw

Beat together 1 tablespoon low calorie salad dressing and 2 tablespoons vegetable oil. Marinate in this 1 medium carrot (roughly grated) and 1 level tablespoon finely grated onion. Add sugar and seasoning to taste. Leave for several hours then, just before serving, add finely shredded cabbage and toss.

Spanish Tomato Salad

Slice 3 or 4 tomatoes thinly. Cut a green pepper into thin rings. Slice 1 large Spanish onion thinly and separate into rings. Mix and dress with oil and cider vinegar.

Waldorf Salad

Line a large, shallow dish with lettuce leaves. Chop and mix equal quantities of celery and red apples. Cover the leaves and top with halved, stoned grapes (or small seedless ones) chopped walnuts and dates.

Cocktail Salad

Diced apple, pineapple, grated orange peel, desiccated coconut, diced orange, melon, tomato. Serve on lettuce and chives with French dressing.

Hawaiian Salad

Small green peas, grapes, sliced lemon, melon, capers, oranges, apples and grated nuts. Serve on a base of lettuce, tomato slices and apple-mint with French dressing or low-calorie salad dressing.

Tropical Salad

Sliced orange, pineapple, grapefruit, chopped celery, olives, chopped walnuts, green peppers. Serve on watercress and mint with a dressing of mayonnaise.

Tomato and Pineapple Salad

Take three or four large firm tomatoes. Cut a slice off the stem end and scoop out the centres. Mix the pulp with tiny cubes of pineapple and chopped parsley. Put the mixture back into tomato cases, and serve in a bed of lettuce with mayonnaise.

Potato Salad

Cook the required amount of potatoes and while they are still hot, skin them and cut them into cubes. Place in a warmed bowl and add a small cooked beetroot, cut up small, for each pound of potatoes. Season with salt, oil and lemon juice. Add some chopped parsley and spring onions and serve while still warm.

Beetroot Salad

Slice a cooked beetroot into lemon juice, sprinkle with brown sugar and chopped fresh mint. Serve with salad greens and Soya Cheese or Tofu.

Salad Hints

Add nuts (whole, grated, flaked or ground), and/or a little fruit, fresh or dried to vegetable salads for variety.

Suitable fresh fruits are chopped apple, sliced orange or banana, slivers of pineapple, washed dates, roughly cut, or seedless raisins. Experiment with new mixtures for added interest.

Quick dressings can be oil and lemon juice, oil and cider vinegar, or a mixture of a low calorie dressing and oil.

When grating raw beetroot add grated cooking apple to improve colour and flavour.

Salads give plenty of opportunity for artistic expression. Serve them attractively displayed on a large dish as a change from a bowl.

Common foods rich in vitamin A include turnip tops, spinach, beet greens, broccoli-tops, kale, red peppers, lettuce, carrots, watercress, green peppers and diminishing amounts in many other vegetables. Some vitamin A is present in the green parts of all plants as carotene is always found in company with chlorophyll, i.e., the darker leaves of the lettuce are richer than the inner ones. Carotene is much better absorbed when fat is taken at the same time; thus salad oil or a knob of fat on broccoli improves its food value.

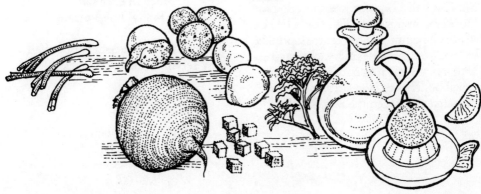

39

Whipped Avocado

Chill fruit. Remove flesh and whip with 3-4 teaspoons of a low calorie salad dressing. Return to shells and serve with green salad.

Avocado and Grapefruit Salad

On a nest of lettuce and watercress arrange alternate slices of avocado and sections of grapefruit (or orange). Garnish with thin strips of red pepper and serve with a dressing of oil and lemon juice.

Quick Avocado Salad

Prepare fresh green salad. Cut avocado in half lengthways. Remove stone but not shell. Sprinkle with lemon juice and eat it from the shell with the salad.

Special Visitor Salad

Put a covering of lettuce leaves on a flat dish. Cut half a skinned ripe avocado pear into 4 lengthways slices. Place on a bed of lettuce all pointing to the centre. Sprinkle well with mayonnaise or French dressing. Put a pineapple ring in the centre and small bunches of land cress or sprigs of watercress between the avocado slices.

Avocado Spread for Sandwiches

Mix the mashed fruit with any sandwich filling or just spread it on bread or dry biscuits. No other fat is necessary.

Mexican 'Dip'

1 Avocado
2 teaspoons lemon juice
Freshly grated onion to taste
Pinch of sea salt
A few sprigs of chopped fresh watercress

1. Mash avocado and stir in the other ingredients. Serve with celery sticks.

Salad Dressings

Mustard and Cress Garni

2 tablespoons lemon juice
1 teaspoon maple syrup
Pinch fine sea salt
Some finely chopped mint

Toss cress in this dressing just before serving. Add to any salad.

Simple Salad Dressing

Beat together 1 tablespoon lemon juice and 2 tablespoons of vegetable oil. This can be flavoured with finely chopped green onions, parsley, mint or other fresh herbs to taste.

Salad Cream

1 tablespoon undiluted concentrated vegetable milk
1 tablespoon vegetable oil
$1/2$ teaspoon raw cane sugar
Good pinch of sea salt
1 tablespoon lemon juice

1. Mix milk, oil, sugar and salt, then quickly beat in lemon juice and whisk well.

2. This cream should be used within two to three days and stored in the refrigerator if possible. It may be flavoured with paprika, ginger, cardamom, curry powder or chopped fresh herbs, if desired, to add variety.

Tofu Mayonnaise

4 oz (120g) silken tofu
up to 1 oz (30ml) water
1 tablespoon of oil
1 tablespoon of vinegar
$1/2$ teaspoon yellow mustard seed
$1/2$ teaspoon sea salt

Put everything in the blender, using less of the water if you require a thicker finish.

Note: If you need to substitute the silken tofu, warm $1^{1}/2$ teaspoons of agar-agar in $1/2$ pt (280ml) of milk and leave to set. Whisk up and use.

French Dressing

2 parts vegetable oil to
1 part cider vinegar
Sea salt

Put all ingredients in a screw-top jar and shake well.

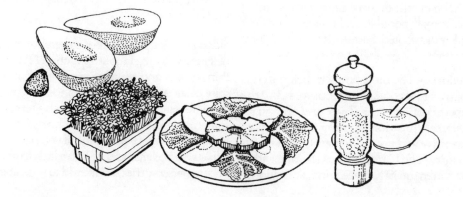

SOME EXOTIC FRUITS AND VEGETABLES

Aubergine — The rich purple of the aubergine — or eggplant — is now a familiar sight in British shops. They are obtainable almost all year round as they are imported from the Canary Islands, East Africa, Israel and the Mediterranean countries. The flavour is distinctive and, as well as making a tasty addition to a main meal — just sliced and lightly fried — they are excellent in ratatouille, goulash, etc.

Fennel — the onion shaped, celery-like stem vegetable, can be eaten raw — finely shredded in salads — or as an ingredient of soup, etc. It comes mostly from France and Italy, and tastes faintly of aniseed.

Jerusalem Artichokes — a home-grown winter vegetable similar in appearance to a small, very knobbly potato, is excellent eaten raw. Crisp, nutty and not at all expensive. Trim carefully and slice or chop, that is all. It is not related to the potato, but a sort of second-cousin-twice-removed to the sunflower. They are not really artichokes and have no connection with Jerusalem.

Courgettes or **Zucchini** — these tiny members of the marrow family are becoming increasingly popular, and therefore are now widely distributed. Slice and fry for 3 minutes or steam as vegetable marrow.

Melon — The most popular melon in this country is, of course, the Honeydew, but the experts consider the Tiger and the Sugar melon are superior. However, they are more expensive and not so frequently seen in this country. The Cantaloupe is the one with a net pattern on its furrowed rind, and reddish-orange flesh. One to try if possible is the French Charentais, small, with pink flesh and a delicate flavour. Or the Ogen, also small, with greenish-yellow flesh and a sweet, strong flavour. This one comes from Israel. Melons are cheapest in August and September. Squash and pumpkin are cooked in some places, but have never been popular here.

Okra — sometimes called **Ladies Fingers**, looks very much like chillies, but they are slimmer and have 5 semi-flattened sides. The ones we see here come from Kenya. These are cooked like courgettes or small marrows, and are good sliced in salads.

Sweet Potatoes — have a pink skin and a slightly more pointed shape than a regular potato, but can be cooked in similar ways. Most of those we get come from the Canary Islands. Scrub and scald then roast in hot oil with a sprinkle of dill seeds for 40 minutes at 425°F/220°C (Gas Mark 7).

Mangetout — The small, almost flat, green peas we sometimes see in January are called mangetout — 'eat whole.' They come from Morocco mostly and are cooked and eaten whole. The peas are almost non-existent, the pods have the flavour, and very good and sweet they are, sliced, raw or very lightly cooked (5 minutes) in ½-inch (1cm) of oil and water.

Salsify — is a winter root vegetable from Belgium. It is long (about 10 inches/125cm), thin, brown and usually very dusty. But in spite of its off-putting appearance it is very good to eat, with a crisp, nutty texture something like a Jerusalem artichoke. Scrub well, scrape or pare very thinly if you have an adjustable peeler, and slice into a little lemon juice to preserve the colour. Add to vegetable salad. Alternatively, fry small chunks in a little oil for 3-5 minutes, and serve with a protein dish.

Capsicum — The capsicum family, of which there are hundreds of members, includes the now popular red and green peppers and chillies. Well known for their very high vitamin C value, they can be bought all year round, for they are imported from quite a few countries. The red peppers are usually a little sweeter than the green, but are usually higher in price. Cayenne pepper is the dried, ground flesh of the capsicum.

Lychees — are usually thought of as a Chinese fruit, but the fresh ones sold in this country from December to February have been grown in South Africa. Round and brown, with a very tough, slightly rough, crisp skin, this white, juicy fruit has a very sweet, distinctive and pleasant flavour. Unfortunately, the price keeps them out of the 'everyday' class.

Pineapples — vary considerably in price according to season. Although available all year round, from one country or another, they are considered to be at their best for flavour in November and December. Our supplies come principally from South Africa, Kenya and the Azores.

In December especially there is a bewildering range of oranges and tangerines in the shops and it is not always easy to remember their individual characteristics. Here are just a few:

Tangerines — have the strongest flavour but many pips. They come from Italy.

Mandarins — also from Italy and **Wilkins** from Morocco, are also rather pippy.

Satsumas — are almost seedless, but

Clementines although they have some pips, are preferable for flavour.

Chestnuts — The best to be found in the greengrocers are Italian. The French ones are ready first, but do not keep so well. We also import from Spain. The dealers in New Covent Garden Market complain that the large Italian chestnuts are scarce because the French people prefer them for their marrons glacés (candied chestnuts).

Limes — when we get them — which is not often — come to us from Kenya, although a great many are grown in the West Indies.

Fresh Dates — It is now possible to get them from time to time. Rather expensive, they are packed in little punnets like strawberries and flown in from Israel. A rare luxury.

Mooli — is a long, thin, white, continental radish. It comes from East Africa and can be sliced and used in salads for a change. Not as attractive as our indigenous red ones though.

Mangoes — A taste for mangoes usually has to be acquired, but the fruit is greatly appreciated by those who have succeeded. Mangoes are invariably associated in our minds with India, but the ones which find their way into our shops have been grown in Africa. They are rather costly in this country, particularly as they have a huge stone. They are ready to eat when not actually hard to touch. Choose as you would avocados.

Batavia — is a lettuce very similar to endive, the leaves of which are equally shaggy but less 'curled'.

Avocado — Nature's Green Butter — Green, pear-shaped and, because it contains up to 25 per cent high quality unsaturated fat and more protein than any other fruit, the avocado can be a valuable addition to any diet. It also contains a good supply of vitamins and minerals. Make sure your avocado is ripe by touch. Hold in the hand and very gently press near the stalk. If the fruit responds slightly it is ripe. If the flesh is firm, keep the avocado at room temperature until it is in perfect condition for eating. Then cut in half, remove the large stone and outer skin (tough enough to afford it ample protection from natural and man-made dangers). The flesh should mash quite easily for sandwich fillings. For salads it should be sliced or diced.

Although we refer to some fruits as being 'acid' — pineapple, all citrus fruits, strawberries, raspberries, etc. — their effect on the system, when eaten, is alkaline.

Ways with Vegetables

Corn on the Cob
(Maize)

This must be carefully timed, for if cooked too long, it becomes tough. Boil in salted water for 8 to (not more than) 12 minutes, according to size and freshness of the cob. A freshly picked cob will cook easily in 8 minutes. Strain, dribble over vegetable oil and serve. Tender young heads can be stripped and the corn eaten raw in salads.

Onions-de-Luxe

1 tablespoon nut butter or vegan margarine
1 lb (445g) smallish onions of equal size
⅓ pint (200ml) grapefruit juice
1 tablespoon brown sugar
1 teaspoon soya flour
2 tablespoons cold water

1. Melt the nut butter in a heavy pan and make sure the bottom and sides are coated.

2. Put the peeled onions in the pan with the fruit juice and sprinkle with sugar. Cover and simmer until tender (about 20 minutes).

3. Remove onions and mix soya flour and water. Add to the onion liquid and cook gently for a few minutes, stirring. Pour over the onions.

Mashed Swedes

1 lb (455g) swedes
Sea salt
1 oz (30g) vegan margarine
Cayenne pepper

1. Peel the swedes thickly if old, thinly if young. Place in a pan, just cover with water, add salt. Bring to the boil, then simmer for 30 minutes or until tender.

2. Drain, beat in margarine and add seasoning to taste.

Sweet Onions

1 medium apple — any kind
2 small onions
1 tablespoon vegetable oil or vegan margarine
2 tablespoons Barbados sugar (or a little more if cooking apple is used).

1. Wash, core and slice the apple — do not skin.

2. Peel and slice the onions and cook in the oil until nearly tender.

3. Add the apple and a little water. Cover and simmer until the apple is cooked — just a few minutes.

4. Sprinkle with the sugar and continue on a very low heat until all the moisture has evaporated.

Leeks

Sea salt and pepper
Lemon juice
Well washed leeks
Vegetable oil
Breadcrumbs

1. Oil a fireproof dish. Sprinkle with salt, pepper and lemon juice. Lay in one row of leeks. If more than this is to be cooked, repeat the oil and seasoning between.

2. Sprinkle wih fresh breadcrumbs and bake in moderate oven 350°F/180°C (Gas Mark 4) for 15 to 20 minutes.

Cabbage

The secret of serving perfect cabbage, etc., is to slightly undercook in a little or no water. Wash and shred cabbage finely. Heat ½ inch (1cm) of oil and water in a pan with well-fitting lid. Toss in cabbage and very little salt. Cover and shake from time to time while cooking, but do not remove the lid. Use low heat. Cooking time is 3-4 minutes. Cabbage should be served while still fairly crisp. This method can be used for all green, leafy vegetables and greatly improves the flavour as well as conserving the nutrients. Use any remaining water in gravy or stock.

Roast Parsnips

Scrub parsnips and skin if necessary. Cut lengthwise to even size and boil for 3 minutes in just enough salted water to cover. Strain and dry over low heat while heating oil in baking tin. Put parsnips in hot oil and turn to cover all sides with oil. Return to hot oven 400°F/200°C (Gas Mark 6) and roast until brown and tender. Approximately 30 minutes. Turn once during cooking. The time needed will depend on the age of the parsnips. Small young ones will cook very quickly. If the oven is not in use, the steamed parsnips can be cooked in a pan on top of the cooker.

The Chinese Way

Pour one tablespoon of oil into heavy (lidded) pan. Scrub vegetables and cut small. Cover and cook very lightly, shaking from time to time, for 3-6 minutes according to vegetables being cooked. Serve immediately, while still firm and crisp. This method retains the flavour and appearance and ensures the minimum loss of vitamins.

Spinach

2 tablespoons vegetable oil
1 small onion (chopped or sliced)
1 lb (455g) spinach
Sea salt

1. Put oil in pan. Add onion and sauté lightly (do not brown).

2. Wash spinach and remove thick stalk. Drain. Chop the spinach and add the onion. Cover the pot and cook gently for 2-3 minutes.

Note: Basic recipe can be varied by adding mushrooms, tomatoes, mint or parsley. If mint is used only a small amount is needed but be generous with the parsley.

Onions in Batter
(Deep Fried)

Peel large onions and slice across into ¼ inch (5mm) thick rings. Have a deep, heavy pan filled only one third with oil, place on medium heat until it reaches 375°F/190°C — no higher. Dip the onion rings in batter and fry for about 2 minutes or until golden. These will be beautifully crisp if correct temperature is maintained.

Do not try to cook a basketful at one time, this will lower the heat, take longer, and not have such good results.

Aubergines

This vegetable has a sweetish, distinctive but very pleasant flavour. It has, however, the unfortunate reputation of being bitter. However, it is only the large or old egg-plants (as they are sometimes known) which may be bitter and this can easily be remedied. If it is suspected of being overgrown, cut the aubergine into thick slices, lightly sprinkle salt on both sides and leave for a few minutes. Blot the slices on kitchen paper and proceed as with a younger vegetable.

Oil both sides of the slices (remove nothing, all is edible) and bake in an uncovered dish at 400°F/200°C (Gas mark 6) for approximately 12 minutes,turning once during this time. Alternatively grill or shallow fry lightly on both sides for a few minutes only. Delicious as they are with any dish, but for variety serve with a lemon butter sauce — beat margarine and add fresh lemon juice slowly, drop by drop.

Lettuce and Peas

Slice a little onion finely, cook for 2 or 3 minutes with a tablespoon of oil, do not brown. Wash and shred several outside leaves of lettuce, stir into the onion, add shelled peas and season, cook slowly with the lid on; do not allow to boil dry.

Jerusalem Artichoke Chips

Trim and thinly slice artichokes and fry in hot oil until brown and crisp.

Vitamins from the Garden

Ring the changes with dandelion leaves, the top leaves of nettles and radish tops. These can all be lightly cooked and served with a savoury dish. All dark green leafy vegetables are rich in vitamins and often calcium also. Cook as spinach.

An alternative way of serving is to chop the cooked vegetables and blend in a little peanut butter or home-made nut cream. Add a small quantity of finely chopped onion and, if liked a few drops of soya sauce.

Make the Most of Your Juices

Lightly steam any vegetables in vegetable juice instead of water. This is not wildly extravagant for well-washed outside leaves of lettuce, cabbage, etc. provide a juice of superior value as they normally contain more colour (chlorophyll, etc.). The flavour of the cooked vegetables as well as the nutritional value is enhanced. Use surplus juice also for cooking whole rice, wheat, lentils, etc., in place of all water if stock is not available. Try cooking pre-soaked butter beans in a mixture of carrot and celery juice, which is delicious. Never discard vegetable water. When there is no immediate use for it in the kitchen, drink it, with a little yeast extract added if liked.

Ways with Potatoes

First — how *not* to cook.

The too common practice of peeling a potato, discarding the skin — together with the most nutritious and tasty part immediately below the skin — boiling it thoroughly, throwing away more of the nutrient in the water, and then mashing it with butter and/or milk is wasteful, foolish, and the very best way to deprive your family of both flavour and vitamin C. Boiled or steamed potatoes can be skinned after cooking without removing flavour or potato.

Baking, frying or boiling potatoes in their skins causes less loss of vitamin C than other methods. Although potatoes are only mediocre sources of this vitamin, because they are frequently and widely used, they are an important source of supply, especially in winter when they account for about one third of the vitamin C content in the British diet.

However, vegetarians usually eat plenty of raw vegetables and fruit, so that they rely on potatoes for only a proportionately small amount of this vitamin.

Mashed potatoes contain hardly any vitamin C and are high in calories, particularly when fat is added. Because of this vitamin C loss, some makes of commercially prepared instant potato now have vitamin C added.

The green patches on potatoes and sprouting potatoes contain a poisonous alkaloid, solanidine, and should not be eaten. Potatoes with blight should also be rejected.

The effect of the starch in potatoes is

lessened if the skins are also eaten.

All vegetables should be plunged into boiling water — or hot oil — to avoid the unnecessary loss of vitamin C. Vitamin E is heat resistant and, like protein, is not harmed by cooking.

JACKET POTATOES

The best way to retain most nutritive value is to bake potatoes in their skins. Choose evenly sized, largish potatoes, one for each person. Scrub scrupulously, clean and trim if necessary. Run a sharp knife round the centre to prevent bursting in the oven. Bake for 40-50 minutes, according to size, with the oven at 400°F/200°C (Gas mark 6). When cooked, hold carefully in cloth and press gently to allow steam to escape. Potatoes should be floury, and skins crisp and tough enough to encourage thorough mastication. Serve with parsley butter.

If skins are too tough for the older person when cooked this way, rub potatoes over with a little oil before baking. This keeps them softer and gives added flavour. Alternatively, after lightly oiling, bake in casserole.

JACKET POTATOES WILL MAKE A MEAL IF STUFFED

1. After cooking remove the centre and mix it with chopped parsley and a little grated raw onion. Return to potato shell. Top with a slice of soya cheese and brown under the grill.
2. Mix cooked potato with grated nuts — Brazils are very good for this — before returning to the jacket.
3. After removing some of the centre of the cooked potato, fill with any left over cooked peas, beans or lentils, return to the potato,

reheat and sprinkle with chopped mint or any other fresh herb preferred.

BROWNED POTATOES

Scrub and trim one large potato per person. Cut into quarters. Warm 2 oz (55g) fat or oil in a flat ovendish, turn potato pieces in this and place in a fairly hot oven 400°F/200°C (Gas mark 6). After 15 minutes remove from heat and pour in ¼ pint (140ml) boiling water and bake for approximately another 45 minutes. Turn potatoes once or twice during this time to get evenly browned.

Note: When frying sliced potatoes, toss in seasoned flour before cooking. They will then brown more quickly.

FROSTED POTATOES

Allow one fairly large potato for each person. Scrub and boil in salted water for 10 minutes. Skin and cut in half lengthways. Dip in seasoned flour, place cut side down in a tin of hot oil. Baste with fat so that all sides of the potatoes are covered. Roast in a hot oven at 450°F/230°C (Gas Mark 8) for 30-35 minutes. Potatoes should be well browned.

Hungarian Potatoes

2 medium-sized onions
Vegetable oil for cooking
Paprika
2 tomatoes
1½ lb (680g) potatoes

1. Slice onions and fry in oil adding a pinch of paprika.

2. Scald, skin and slice tomatoes and add to the onions and mix.

3. Slice the potatoes rather thickly and add to the onions and tomatoes. Pour over sufficient water or stock to just cover.

4. Cook slowly in the oven at 375°F/190°C (Gas Mark 5) for 45 minutes until the stock is absorbed, sprinkle with chopped parsley before serving.

Crumbed Potatoes

1½ lb (680g) potatoes
2 oz (55g) oil
2 oz (55g) fresh breadcrumbs
Seasoning

1. Scrub potaoes and cut into thick slices. Cover with boiling water and stand for 3 minutes only. Drain.

2. Heat fat in a large roasting tin, add potato slices. Sprinkle with fresh breadcrumbs and bake at 400°F/200°C (Gas Mark 6) until brown and crisp for 40-50 minutes.

Roasting

1 lb (455g) potatoes
About 4 tablespoons vegetable oil

1. Well scrub potatoes, cut into evenly sized pieces. Heat oil in roasting tin in oven. Dry potatoes and turn in hot oil until all sides have been coated.

2. Roast for 50-60 minutes with oven at 425°F/220°C (Gas Mark 7), according to size of pieces. Turn once or twice during cooking. Lightly sprinkle with salt and remove from oil as soon as browned.

Potato Boats

Allow one large potato per person. Scrub and boil gently in their skins until only just cooked, lay on their sides. Cut a little off the top lengthways and scoop out the centre. Dice and mix with any available cooked vegetable, some chopped mint or parsley and some white sauce. Fill the 'boats' with this mixture and cover with a slice of tomato and brown under the grill.

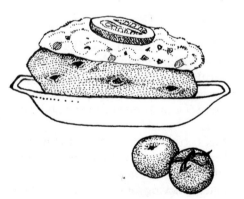

Golden Potatoes

A new way with new potatoes. Choose smallish potatoes which will just cover the base of a saucepan. Pour over just enough oil to come about half-way up the potatoes. Add enough water to bring the liquid up to cover them. Bring quickly to boil, without covering, and keep boiling steadily until all the water has evaporated.

Turn potatoes so that both sides get brown and do not allow them to stick to the pan. Remove and strain off any oil left in the pan, and sprinkle with chopped parsley. Cooking time approximately 20 minutes.

Potato Bake

Mashed potato
Garlic or vegetable salt
Sliced onions and tomatoes fried together.

1. Place half the mashed potato in a greased pie dish, cover with the tomato and onion mixture and top with the rest of the potato.

2. Reheat in the oven or brown under the grill for a few minutes. Serve with gravy, a green vegetable and a protein dish such as nut rissoles.

Thymed Potatoes

1 lb (455g) potatoes
2 tablespoons vegetable oil
1 onion, chopped
7oz (200g) tomatoes, skinned
1 teaspoon thyme
Seasoning

Scrub potaoes well and cut into small dice. Heat oil in saucepan, add potatoes and onion. When lightly browned, add tomatoes, thyme and seasoning. Cook for about 20 minutes, until just tender.

Bircher Potatoes

Scrub and thickly slice potatoes. Place in well-oiled shallow tin, sprinkle with caraway seeds and a little salt. Bake for 30 minutes at 400°F/200°C (Gas Mark 6). The potatoes should be brown and crispy. Some say that caraway seeds aid digestion, in any case they taste very good.

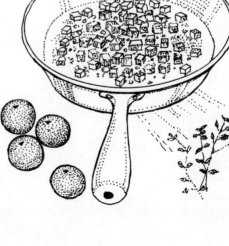

Savoury Potatoes I

1½ lb (680g) potatoes
3 tablespoons oil
1 large onion
1 teaspoon sage
Seasoning
1 tablespoon water

1. Thinly peel potatoes and cut in half.

2. Oil an ovenproof casserole dish. Put a layer of onions in the bottom of the dish, add potatoes cut side down, sprinkle with more chopped onions, sage and seasoning.

3. Top with the rest of the oil and water. Cover and bake in a hot oven 375°F/190°C (Gas Mark 5) for 1 hour. Remove lid and allow potatoes to brown for a further 10 minutes or so.

Savoury Potatoes II

Oven 300°F/150°C (Gas Mark 2). Cooking time 1¾ hours. Scrub and thickly slice the potatoes. Place in oiled casserole and sprinkle with grated onion and finely chopped mushrooms. Cover with stock, replace lid and bake.

Scalloped Potatoes

Oil a casserole. Slice scrubbed potatoes very thinly. Place in casserole in layers with any other vegetables in season or to hand: celery, onion, carrot, etc. Mix enough vegetable oil with double quantity of stock to just cover the vegetables. Bake for 1 hour at 350°F/180°C (Gas Mark 4) in covered dish. Remove lid for the last 10 minutes to brown the top.

MAIN MEALS

When planning meals, remember that, to be appreciated, roasts, soups and rissoles should contain at least one of the most flavoursome vegetables, i.e., onions, leeks, garlic, aubergines, mushrooms, celery or tomatoes. Natural and beneficial savoury flavourings which can be added if necessary are yeast extract, soy sauce or any of the herbs in small quantities. Spices, on the other hand, should be used very sparingly.

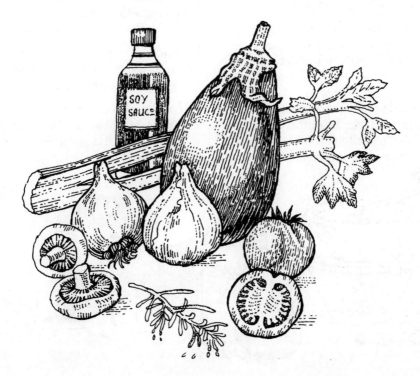

Basic Nutmeat Mixture

1 medium onion
¼ pint (140ml) vegetable stock
4 oz (115g) milled mixed nuts
1 oz (30g) muesli base
2 level teaspoons soya flour
2 teaspoons vegetable oil
½ teaspoon mixed herbs
1 level teaspoon yeast extract

1. Chop onion finely and simmer in stock for 5-10 minutes.

2. Mix all ingredients together with the vegetable stock to stiffish consistency. Put into greased basin and cover with greaseproof paper.

3. Steam for 1½ hours, or bake in an oven-proof dish for 30 minutes at 350°F/180°C (Gas Mark 4).

Variation

Add mushrooms, or tomatoes, or fill with chestnut stuffing. This mixture may also be used to stuff marrows, aubergines, green peppers, tomatoes, etc.

Stuffed Butter Bean Roast

4oz (115g) butter beans
1 medium onion (4 oz/115g)
2oz (55g) wholemeal breadcrumbs
1 teaspoon soya flour
Seasoning
½ teaspoon sage
1 large tomato

1. Soak butter beans overnight. Remove outer skin. Simmer until soft (allow 50 minutes). Drain and pass through sieve or mash.

2. Chop onion and fry lightly.

3. Mix beans, breadcrumbs, soya flour, seasoning and onion together, form into roll. Cut through centre.

4. Place thick slices of tomato on one half. Replace the other half of roll, cover with greased paper.

5. Bake in fairly hot oven (400°F/200°C, Gas mark 6) for about 20 minutes. Serve with gravy and green vegetables.

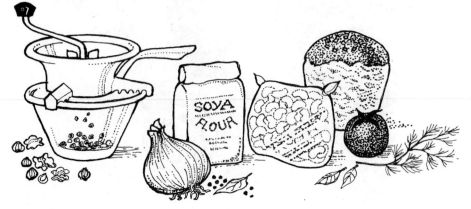

CURRIED TEXTURED VEGETABLE PROTEIN

1½ oz (45g) unflavoured textured
vegetable protein, mince or chunks
8 fl oz (230ml) stock or water
1 onion, chopped (about 3oz/85g)
2 tablespoons vegetable oil
2 teaspoons curry powder
2 teaspoons lime or lemon juice
1 small apple, chopped
1 teaspoon coconut (optional)
Sea salt
1 oz (30g) seedless raisins
2 teaspoons tomato ketchup
2 cloves
A few cooked chestnuts

1. Simmer the mince in stock for 10
minutes (if chunks are used allow 15-20
minutes).

2. Sauté the onion in the oil for 10
minutes. Gradually sprinkle in the curry
powder, stirring all the time until quite
smooth. Cook for a few more minutes
then add lemon juice and the rest of the
ingredients.

3. Stir in the textured vegetable protein
and simmer, covered, very gently for at
least 20 minutes. Serve on a bed of rice.

STUFFED MARROW

4 oz (115g) lentils
1 small onion
¼ pint (140ml) stock
1oz (30g) fresh breadcrumbs
1 teaspoon agar agar
½ teaspoon dried sage
Lemon juice
2 tablespoons vegetable oil
Seasoning

1. Cook lentils and chopped onion in
stock for 20 minutes, keeping pan covered.

2. Add more water if necessary. Stir in
breadcrumbs and agar (which has been
dissolved in a little water), herbs, lemon
juice, oil and seasoning.

3. Cut marrow in half lengthways amd
remove seeds. Do not peel. Place in baking
tin with a little oil, cover with greased
paper and bake at 300°F/150°C (Gas
Mark 2) for 30 minutes.

4. Fill with the stuffing and return to oven
for another 30 minutes, raising the heat
for the last 10 minutes to brown.

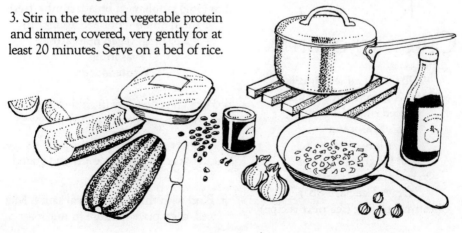

Brazil and Walnut Basic Mixture

2-3 oz (55-85g) chopped onions
2 oz (30g) vegetable oil
1 teaspoon sage
1 teaspoon dried basil
1/4 teaspoon sea salt
1 good teaspoon yeast extract
8 fl oz (220ml) hot water
6 oz (170g) wholemeal breadcrumbs
1 oz (30g) wholemeal flour
1 oz (30g) soya flour
3 oz (85g) milled Brazil nuts
3 oz (85g) chopped walnuts

1. Cook chopped onion in the oil.

2. Add the herbs, salt, yeast extract and hot water. Then the breadcrumbs. Allow to stand for a few minutes.

3. Mix flour and soya and stir into nuts. Add to the onion mixture and mix until smooth.

Brazil Nut Roast with Chestnut Stuffing

1/2 lb (225g) milled Brazils
6 oz (170g) fresh breadcrumbs
Grated rind of 1 lemon
Seasoning
1 large onion
2 oz (55g) vegetable oil
1/2 teaspoon powdered sage
Gravy (see page 88)
Chestnut stuffing (see next recipe)

1. Mix the nuts, breadcrumbs, lemon rind and seasoning.

2. Cut onion and cook lightly in oil, add sage.

3. Add onion to crumb mixture, and enough gravy or vegetable stock to make a stiff roll.

4. Press half the mixture into a greased bread tin, cover with Chestnut Stuffing. Add the rest of the mixture.

5. Cover with greased paper and cook in fairly hot oven 400°F/200°C (Gas Mark 6) for about 30 minutes. Garnish with tomatoes and parsley.

Variation: Potato Pie
Put the nut mixture into a greased oven-proof dish, cover with a few slices of lightly fried, thick slices of tomato or aubergine. Top with mashed potatoes and brown under the grill.

Chestnut Stuffing I

1 lb (455g) chestnuts
1 tablespoon chopped parsley
2 oz (55g) wholemeal breadcrumbs (fresh)
1 small onion (chopped and fried)
2 oz (55g) vegan margarine
Seasoning
White sauce

1. Place the chestnuts in cold water, bring to the boil, peel and boil until cooked.

2. Mash or press the nuts through a sieve, add parsley, crumbs, onion and grated margarine.

3. Bind with thick wholemeal sauce. Mix well, then place mixture in nut roast.

CHESTNUT CRISPIES

Using the same mixture, form into small balls, roll in fresh breadcrumbs and bake in hot oven for a few minutes. It will make them beautifully crisp on the outside. Serve with any savoury roast.

COOKING CHESTNUTS
Alternative Method

Cover with cold water and bring to the boil. Remove from the heat and leave in the water — keeping it hot — for 20 minutes. Take only two or three at a time from the water when the skins can be easily removed. If chestnuts are to be passed through a sieve for use in stuffing, etc. they may require a little longer in the water.

GRANDAD'S SHEPHERDS PIE

2½ oz (70g) tvp mince
1 largish onion
2 teaspoons vegetable oil
½ oz (15g) wholemeal flour
1 teaspoon yeast extract
¼ pint (140ml) vegetable stock
1 tablespoon tomato ketchup
1 lb (455g) potatoes, cooked and mashed

1. Soak the mince in water for 10 minutes. Meanwhile gently fry the onion in oil. Add the flour to the onions and cook for a further few minutes.

2. Add the yeast extract and some of the stock and stir until the mixture thickens. Stir in the ketchup and any seasoning desired. If necessary, add the rest of the stock, but the mixture should not be very moist.

3. Strain off the mince and add to the savoury mixture. Turn into a pie dish and cover with the mashed potato. Cook at 350°F/180°C (Gas Mark 4) for 30 minutes or until nicely browned.

ECONOMY CASSEROLE

2 oz (55g) celery
4 oz (115g) carrots
4 oz (115g) parsnips
6 oz (170g) leeks
4 oz (115g) cooked brown rice
1 large tomato or aubergine
½ pint (285ml) vegetable stock or water
1 teaspoon yeast extract
1 teaspoon soya flour mixed with
1 heaped teaspoon flaked millet
A good handful of parsley

1. Chop and fry the vegetables in a little oil for 5 minutes.

2. Place vegetables and rice in casserole. Top with slices of tomato or aubergine.

3. Pour over the water or stock in which the yeast extract has been dissolved. Sprinkle over millet and crisp under the grill. Serve with a green vegetable.

Brazil and Hazelnut Roast

2 oz (55g) Brazils
1 oz (30g) hazel nuts
1 tablespoon wheat flakes
6 oz (170g) onions — chopped and cooked in 2 tablespoons oil
1 tomato, skinned and chopped
1 teaspoon yeast extract
Pinch of sage
Small handful chopped parsley

Mix and blend ingredients. Oil baking tin and roast mixture for 30 minutes at 375°F/190°C (Gas Mark 5).

Brown Rice and Vegetables

4 oz (115g) cooked brown rice
¾ pint (425ml) water
1 medium onion, chopped and fried
½ lb (225g) tomatoes
2 oz (55g) chopped nuts
2 oz (55g) wholemeal breadcrumbs

1. Wash and boil rice in the water for 10 to 15 minutes. Turn to a very low heat and simmer slowly until cooked — about 20 minutes. Add more water or stock if necessary, but liquid should be absorbed when rice is cooked. (The rice can be cooked the previous day).

2. Place cooked onions in pie dish, add a layer of cooked rice, a layer of thickly sliced tomatoes, sprinkle over with nuts and cover with breadcrumbs.

3. Bake in a fairly hot oven 400°F/200°C (Gas Mark 6) for 30 minutes.

4. Wholewheat can be used in place of rice for a change. When no nuts are handy, this gives a fine nutty consistency. Many variations can be concocted with the basic cooked rice or wheat, onions, tomatoes and nuts. Add mushrooms, thinly sliced carrot or other root vegetable, or celery, to the onions while cooking. Or add a good teaspoon of soy sauce for added flavour.

Savoury Nut Roll

3½ oz (100g) white fat
½ lb (225g) wholemeal flour
¼ pint (140ml) water
1 teaspoon yeast extract
1 small fried onion
1 small fried leek
4 oz (115g) millet nuts
1 small grated carrot
Parsley
A pinch of sweet basil

1. Blend together fat, flour and water then roll into an oblong shape.

2. Spread the pastry with the yeast extract and cover with the onion and the leek.

3. Sprinkle on the milled nuts and lastly the grated carrot and herbs. Roll up carefully, seal the edges and prick the top.

4. Bake at 400°F/200°C (Gas Mark 6), for 30 minutes. Serve with Gravy (see page 88) and green vegetables.

Mushroom and Cashew Nut Pie

½ lb (225g) cashew nuts
½ pint (285ml) vegetable stock or water
1 onion, medium size
2 oz (55g) vegan margarine
1 teaspoon thyme or marjoram
½ lb (225g) mushrooms
1 tablespoon wholemeal flour
½ teaspoon yeast extract
Sea salt

For short-crust pastry:
3 oz (85g) white fat
6 oz (170g) wholemeal flour (plain)
1 tablespoon cold water

1. Soak the cashew nuts in the water or stock overnight.

2. Peel and chop the onion and cook gently in the fat with the herbs for 10 minutes.

3. Add the mushrooms, washed and roughly chopped, and cook for 5 minutes. Stir in the flour and the nuts with their water. Cover and simmer for 30 minutes.

4. To make the pastry rub the fat into the flour until the mixture resembles breadcrumbs. Add the cold water and gather mixture together to form a ball. Roll out to the desired shape (this is easily and cleanly done between layers of greaseproof paper).

5. Add the yeast extract and salt to the mushroom and cashew nut mixture. Put into a pie dish and allow to cool before covering with pastry and baking at 400°F/200°C (Gas Mark 6) for 30 minutes. Serve with lightly cooked vegetables.

Bean Layer Pie

6 oz (170g) beans (black-eyed beans are good for this)
1 large onion (chopped)
2 tablespoons vegetable oil
3 medium tomatoes (skinned)
2 sticks celery (sliced)
1 small green pepper (deseeded and chopped)
Seasoning
1 tablespoon chopped fresh parsley or
1 teaspoon other dried herbs

1. Cook beans in double the quantity of water for about 30 minutes.

2. Fry onion in the oil for a few minutes then add tomatoes, celery and pepper. Cook together for about 5 minutes.

3. Place layers of beans and vegetables in an oiled oven-proof dish adding seasoning and herbs to taste.

4. Cover with mashed potato and bake in a moderate oven 325°F/170°C (Gas Mark 3) for about 30 minutes.

5. Serve with lightly cooked juicy green vegetable such as cabbage or kale.

Individual Pies with Nut Pastry

For Filling:
1 oz (30g) tvp mince
1 onion (about 6 oz/170g), chopped
Vegetable oil for cooking
1 carrot (about 4 oz/115g), diced
Green peas (about 4 oz/115g)
Gravy (see page 88)
½ teaspoon yeast extract

For Pastry:
A good 2 oz (55g) vegan margarine
2 oz (55g) wholemeal flour
2½ oz (70g) 81% flour
1½ oz (45g) ground Brazil nuts
Cold water to mix, a little less than
2 tablespoons

1. Soak tvp in hot water for 5-10 minutes. Strain off any surplus water and gently cook onions and tvp in a little oil for 10 minutes.

2. Cook carrots and peas for a few minutes then add to the tvp onion mixture.

3. Add the gravy mix and yeast extract to taste.

4. Make the pastry by rubbing the margarine into the flour and Brazil nuts, make into a dough with just sufficient cold water.

5. Roll out and line small, deep baking tins (or one for 4 portions), fill with the mixed vegetables, moisten with a little gravy and cover with a pastry lid.

6. Bake at 400°F/200°C (Gas Mark 6) for 30 minutes. To vary these pies, other vegetables can be substituted, or herbs or curry powder can be added.

TVP Marengo

Half packet tvp chunks
Brown stock paste
Vegetable oil
4 oz (115g) chopped mushrooms
½ (285ml) pint vegetable stock
1 crushed clove garlic
1 heaped teaspoon wholemeal flour
2 chopped tomatoes
¼ pint (140ml) white wine (optional)
1 tablespoon tomato purée
Seasoning

1. Soak chunks in water or stock for 15-20 minutes. Bring slowly to the boil, then drain.

2. Toss in the brown stock paste then brown in hot oil and keep warm.

3. Simmer mushrooms in stock for 5 minutes using the pan and hot oil in which the tvp has been cooked, then add the garlic and flour.

4. Add tomatoes and wine. Simmer 15 minutes to reduce liquid.

5. Add tomato purée, season to taste and pour sauce over the chunks.

Suggested accompanying vegetables: Roast potatoes and parsnips.

Rice Pilaff

2 tablespoons vegetable oil
2 medium onions
4 oz (115g) cooked brown rice
2 teaspoons lemon juice
½ teaspoon curry powder
½ pint (285ml) vegetable stock
5 oz (140g) sweetcorn
Seasoning
1 tomato, skinned and chopped
1 red pepper, sliced finely
2 oz (55g) peanuts

1. Heat oil in a heavy pan and cook onion for 5 minutes.

2. Add rice, lemon juice, curry powder, stock, sweetcorn and seasoning. Simmer, covered, for about 20 minutes.

3. Add tomato and a few thin strips of red pepper and cook gently for another 10 minutes, by which time all the liquid should have been absorbed. Stir and add more stock or water if necessary.

4. Add nuts and serve with a good dark green vegetable, such as broccoli or turnip tops.

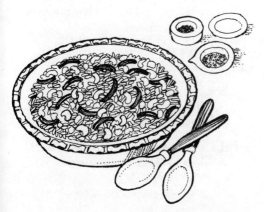

Cooking Rice

Add 2oz (55g/2 rounded tablespoons) brown rice to ½ pint (285ml) of water or vegetable stock and pinch of sea salt. Boil for 20 minutes, reduce heat and simmer very gently, covered, for another 10-20 minutes. By this time all the water should be absorbed and the rice cooked. It will now weigh approximately 4-5 oz (115-140g). If required for a savoury dish, a bay leaf or another herb could be added to the cooking water.

Paella

3 oz (85g) mushrooms, sliced
Vegetable oil for frying
5 oz (140g) brown rice
½ pint (285ml) unsweetened pineapple juice
½ pint (285ml) water
2 tablespoons tomato ketchup
2 oz (55g) sultanas
Half a small green pepper, chopped
2 oz (55g) nuts
Pineapple rings to garnish

1. Sauté the sliced mushrooms in a little oil in a large pan. Then add the rice and cook for a few minutes.

2. Add pineapple juice, ½ pint water and tomato ketchup. Simmer for approx 25-30 minutes until all the liquid is absorbed and the rice tender.

3. Add the sultanas, green pepper and coarsely grated nuts. Heat through and pile into serving dish, surrounded with pineapple rings.

MUSHROOM PIE

4 oz (115g) onions, chopped
2 tablespoons vegetable oil for frying
2 medium tomatoes
1 teaspoon basil or marjoram
4 oz (115g) field mushrooms, sliced
4 oz (115g) cooked brown rice or wheat
A little finely chopped celery (optional)
1 teaspoon soya flour
Seasoning

For Topping:

About 10 oz (285g) potatoes, cooked and
mashed with 1 oz (30g) vegan margarine

1. Fry onions in oil until lightly browned
then add the tomatoes, herbs,
mushrooms, rice and celery, if used.

2. Mix the soya flour with 1 tablespoon of
cold water and stir into the mixture. Add
seasoning then cover and cook gently for
5 minutes: turn into a baking dish, cover
with the mashed potato and brown under
the grill.

3. Serve with a brown gravy and green
vegetables.

RAW NUT
SAVOURY PUDDING

1 large tomato
1 tablespoon vegetable oil
1 small onion, finely grated
3 oz (85g) wholemeal breadcrumbs
4 oz (115g) milled nuts, of any kind or
mixed
Herbs for seasoning

1. Blanch and peel tomato and either
liquidize it in an electric blender or pass
through a sieve into a mixing bowl.

2. Add oil, onion and breadcrumbs, and
thoroughly mix to moisten, then add nuts
and herbs, and blend well.

3. Using a small basin well greased with
margarine, press in the mixture and
smooth down level.

4. Cover it and weight the basin down,
after which it will easily cut into slices for
serving with salad.

SWEETCORN PASTIES

½ lb (225g) onions
1 small potato
corn oil, for cooking
3 tablespoons sweetcorn (cooked)
1 teaspoon yeast extract
4 oz (115g) ground cashews
1 quantity shortcrust pastry
(see page 111)

1. Chop onions finely and slice potatoes
thinly. Cook both in the oil.

2. Add sweetcorn and cook a few minutes
more.

3. Add yeast extract, remove from heat,
add cashews and mix well. Allow to cool.

4. Roll out prepared pastry, cut into 3
circles, fill with the cooked mixture, fold
over and seal using a little water.

5. Bake in the oven at 400°F/200°C (Gas
Mark 6) for 20-25 minutes.

Fricassee with Mushrooms

Generous ½ pint (285ml) stock
2 oz (55g) tvp mince
4 oz (115g) mushrooms, washed and
sliced
3 fl oz (90ml) vegetable oil
1 oz (30g) wholemeal flour
½ pint (285ml) water
Seasoning
Lemon juice
Fresh parsley, chopped

1. Make stock according to the instructions on container, heat and add the tvp to soak.

2. Cook the mushrooms in oil for 5 minutes, add the flour while stirring then add the water gradually. Bring to the boil and allow to thicken, still stirring.

3. Strain and add the tvp, bring back to the boil, season and add lemon juice to taste.

4. Just before serving garnish with chopped parsley. Serve with croûtons of fried bread or broken crispbreads and green vegetables.

Risotto

2 tablespoons vegetable oil
1 onion, chopped
5 oz (140g) brown rice
1 level teaspoon yeast extract
Pinch of any herbs to taste
A little less than ¾ pint (425ml) water
½ lb (225g) mushrooms
1 oz (30g) germinated sunflower seeds (or
other), just beginning to sprout
½ a small red pepper, chopped

1. Heat oil and lightly fry onion. Add rice and cook for a couple of minutes, stirring.

2. Dissolve yeast extract in hot water and add with the herbs before stirring in the water. Simmer gently for 20 minutes.

3. Add mushrooms and continue to cook until rice is ready.

4. Season then add the seeds and chopped pepper.

Baked Savoury Roll

Wholemeal pastry made with ½ lb (225g) flour (see page 110 for method).

For Filling:
4 oz (115g) mixed ground nuts
1 level teaspoon yeast extract
2 medium carrots, grated
1 teaspoon dried basil

1. Roll out the pastry to a rectangular shape, not too thick.

2. Spread thinly with the yeast extract, then the carrots, a light sprinkle of basil (or other herb to taste) and the ground nuts.

3. Roll up and seal the end and the edges and bake in a moderately hot oven 375°F/190°C (Gas Mark 5) for 30 minutes.

4. Serve hot with fresh vegetables, dark greens if possible, and gravy or cold with salad.

Non-steak Savoury Pudding

For Filling:
1 level teaspoon yeast extract
2 oz (55g) tvp (unflavoured)
1 large or 2 small carrots
1 large or 2 small leeks (other root vegetables could be used)
About 4 tablespoons vegetable oil for cooking
1 or 2 tomatoes
Few mushrooms
2 teaspoons commercial gravy mix in a little water

For the Pastry:
½ teaspoon salt
½ lb (225g) self-raising flour (wholemeal or 81%)
3 oz (85g) vegetable suet mixed
Water

Make the stock with the yeast extract and about ½ pint (285ml) hot water (in which other vegetables have been cooked if possible). Add the tvp which will absorb some of the flavour as it absorbs the liquid.

Meanwhile thinly slice the root vegetables and fry lightly in a saucepan with the oil. Remove after a few minutes and put the tomatoes and mushrooms in the oil to cook. This is the basis for a very tasty gravy. Strain the tvp and use ¼ pint of the stock to mix the gravy powder. Stir this into the vegetable flavoured oil and cook, adding more stock if necessary (rather more gravy is required than would be used in a 'meat' pudding). Season to taste.

For the Pastry:
1. Sift the salt with the flour, stir in the suet and mix with about 4 tablespoons water.

2. Roll out fairly thinly and line a pudding basin (approx 5 inches/14cm deep). Fill with the vegetables and vegetable meat and top up with gravy.*

3. Cover with the remainder of the pastry, seal the edges and cook well in a large pan half full of boiling water for not less than one hour. It must not go off the boil.

4. Serve with green vegetables and potatoes.

*Keep any surplus gravy and serve with the pudding.

CRISP ONION RINGS

Peel a large Spanish onion and slice it crosswise into fairly thin rings. Blot on kitchen paper, toss in seasoned wholemeal flour and deep fry in hot oil. Strain and serve immediately.

VEGETABLE GOULASH

½ lb (225g) mushrooms
2 large onions
Vegetable oil, for cooking
Seasoning
Caraway seeds
1 small tin savoury cuts
Tomato sauce or tomato purée,
according to taste
Paprika

1. Wash and slice mushrooms, peel and slice onions. Cook slowly in oil, adding seasoning as desired and a few caraway seeds, but do not brown.

2. Drain gravy from savoury cuts and cut these into small pieces.

3. Fry them separately in oil and then add to the onions and mushrooms with the gravy, some tomato sauce (or purée) and a little paprika. A little water may be needed to make the dish reasonably moist.

4. Cook slowly (in a double saucepan if available) for about ½ hour.

5. A few peas may be added before serving if liked. Top with rings of fried pineapple for a special meal. Serve with roast potatoes and a side plate of lettuce.

LENTIL HOT POT

1½ lb (680g) potatoes, sliced
3 onions, sliced
½ lb (225g) red lentils
Seasoning
1 teaspoon dried herbs, to taste
2 level teaspoons yeast extract
About ¾ pint (425ml) warm water
3-4 tablespoons vegetable oil

1. Into a greased oven-proof dish place layers of potatoes, onions, lentils and herbs, finishing with potatoes.

2. Dissolve yeast extract in warm water and pour over.

3. Pour oil over all and bake for about 1 hour in moderate oven — 325°F/170°C (Gas Mark 3).

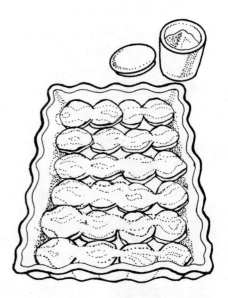

Spaghetti Bolognese

3 oz (85g) tvp mince
1 small onion, chopped
1 stick celery (optional)
1 carrot, chopped
2 tablespoons vegetable oil
1 bay leaf
Pinch of basil (or preferred herb)
1 teaspoon yeast extract
2 tablespoons tomato purée
8 oz (225g) wholemeal spaghetti

1. Leave tvp mince in ½ pint (285ml) water to soak.

2. Lightly fry vegetables in the oil, then strain mince and add to the vegetables with the bay leaf, tomato, basil, yeast extract and tomato purée. Simmer gently for about 30 minutes.

3. Meanwhile, cook spaghetti according to instructions on packet.

4. Remove bay leaf, season and pour over the spaghetti.

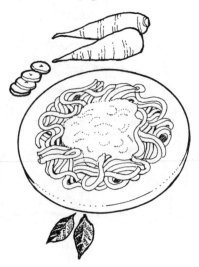

Festive Dinner
(As featured on the BBC programme 'Pebble Mill'.)

Melon and Grapefruit Appetizer

Savoury Steak
— textured vegetable protein dish with tomatoes, chestnuts, grilled pineapple amd rich brown gravy.

Rice Risotto
— with onions, herbs, corn and peas.

Brussels Sprouts
— with white sauce and parsley.

Mixed Salad

Open Mince Tart
— with vegan cream.

Biscuits and Soya Cheese

Recipes

Savoury Steak
— For this we use tvp slices.

Cover tvp meat with plenty of cold water, bring slowly to the boil, simmer for a couple of minutes, then strain.
Press to remove as much liquid as possible, return to the pan and sprinkle liberally with soy sauce, turning so that the flavouring is evenly absorbed. Shallow fry in oil just sufficiently to brown lightly. Be careful not to toughen by over-cooking at this stage. Top with grilled tomatoes and pineapple just before serving.

Rich Brown Gravy

— To the flavoured oil remaining in the pan after browning the Savoury Steak, add flour, stock, browning and seasoning. Pour into gravy boat. (Good gravies and sauces are important when preparing meals for those accustomed to more highly flavoured dishes).

The Chestnuts

— can be prepared at any convenient time, even the day before. Wash, cover with cold water and bring to the boil. Simmer for 20-30 minutes. Strain and re-cover with warm water. Remove the chestnuts one at a time — the skins are easily removed while wet.

White Sauce

— For five-minute sprouts. Ingredients are 1 fl oz (30ml) oil, 1 oz (30g) flour (wholemeal or 81%), 1/4 pint (140ml) concentrated vegetable milk diluted with 1/2 pint (285ml) water and seasoning to taste. Mix the oil and flour in the pan and cook over a very low heat for several minutes, stirring. Add the liquid gradually until the sauce is smooth and creamy. Season. Pour over hot vegetables. (The basic sauce can be flavoured with fresh herbs, onions or even spices if used sparingly.)

Rice Risotto

— To cooked brown rice add some fried onion, a pinch of sage, and mushrooms.

Open Mince Tart

— Make a shortcrust pastry with 1/2 lb (225g) 81% wholemeal flour, 4 oz (115g) white fat (or 3 fl oz (115ml) vegetable oil) and just sufficient very cold water to bind (3-4 tablespoons).

Roll out and cover an 8-9 inch (20-23cm) pie plate with the pastry and fill generously with home-made mincemeat.

Lay a lattice of pastry strips over the fruit and bake at 400°F/200°C (Gas Mark 6) for 30 minutes. If the mincemeat is on the dry side it is as well to cover the tart while cooking until the last few minutes.

Pease Pudding with Corn and Sauce

Clean and dice 6 oz (170g) carrots. Cook over a low heat in a little vegetable oil until tender. Then add a pinch of salt and 1 tablespoon chopped mint (or rather less if dried mint is used). Drain a small tin of sweetcorn and a large tin of pease pudding. Form all ingredients into a loaf, brush with oil and bake for 45 minutes at 375°F/190°C (Gas Mark 5). Garnish with fried onion rings and serve with a green vegetable and sauce. For the sauce, add sufficient water to sweetcorn liquid to make 1/2 pint and bring to boil. Mix one tablespoon of wholemeal flour and soya flour with a little cold water. Add boiling liquid and one teaspoon yeast extract, stir, return to pan and stir until it boils.

Savoury Lentil Purée

½ lb (225g) red lentils
1 small onion, chopped
1 pint (570ml) water or vegetable stock
1 teaspoon yeast extract
1 tablespoon vegetable oil
1 teaspoon lovage or sage

1. Mix lentils, onions and water or stock and cook gently on a low heat for about 20 minutes or until soft.

2. Add yeast extract, oil and herbs. Stir frequently. Water should all be absorbed when ready.

Bengal Curry

2 oz tvp (unflavoured)
1 teaspoon soya sauce
2 fl oz (60ml) vegetable oil
2 medium onions
1 clove garlic (optional)
3 level teaspoons curry powder (more for a hotter flavour)
1 bay leaf
4 tablespoons tomato juice
1 oz (30g) chopped creamed coconut
1 small apple
1 oz (30g) sultanas
A little chopped green ginger
1 teaspoon lemon juice
4 cloves
Seasoning

1. Bring the soya meat to the boil in plenty of water. Strain and press out as much liquid as possible. Add soy sauce and then lightly fry in a little oil, put aside.

2. Skin, chop and fry the onions (and garlic if used) in the rest of the oil. Add curry powder and the bay leaf and simmer gently for a few minutes.

3. Add tomato juice, vegetable meat, coconut, diced apple, sultanas, ginger, lemon juice, cloves (if used) and seasoning. Continue to simmer for a few minutes, remove bay leaf and serve with brown rice and peas or sweetcorn.

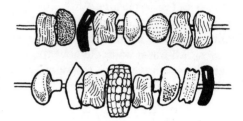

Party Specials: Kebabs

Dissolve 1 stock cube in ½ pint (285ml) red wine (or wine and water). Add a thinly sliced lemon, a small bunch of parsley, and as many tvp chunks as required. Leave to soak for at least 5 minutes. Bring slowly to the boil and simmer for several minutes.

Remove chunks, drain and thread onto kebab skewer with any vegetable to hand: mushroom, tomato, green pepper, cucumber, pineapple, etc. Brush with oil and brown under grill.

Alternatively, serve chunks as buffet snacks. After simmering drain, toss in flour and brown in hot oil. Tvp slices can be used in either of these party recipes.

Vegetable Dishes

When the ingredients in these vegetable dishes do not include a good source of protein, it is advisable to ensure that protein is included elsewhere in the meal. For instance, the dish could be preceded by a soup containing pease pudding, lentils or nut cream, or it could be followed by a salad of fruit and nuts. Or soaked wholewheat or sprouted grains could be served with the savoury — or included in the dish with the other ingredients.

Baked Chestnut Savoury

1 1/2 lb (680g) chestnuts
1 level teaspoon yeast extract
2 large onions
1 tablespoon vegetable oil
1/2 teaspoon sage
1 lb (455g) tomatoes
2 tablespoons wholemeal breadcrumbs or muesli base
1 oz (30g) vegan margarine

1. Cook skinned chestnuts gently with a very little water and the yeast extract, for about 15 minutes.

2. Cut onions into rings and fry until golden brown in the oil, add sage.

3. Place alternate layers of sage and onion, chestnut and sliced tomatoes in oven-proof dish.

4. Lastly, sprinkle over the breadcrumbs and dot with margarine. Bake for 30 minutes at 350°F/180°C (Gas Mark 4).

Potato Hot Pot

Shallots or onion, chopped
Carrots, scrubbed and cut very small
Celery, washed and cut across very thinly
Vegetable oil for frying
Potatoes steamed in skins, then skinned and diced
Celery seed
Vegetable stock

1. Fry vegetables, other than potatoes, lightly in oil.

2. Turn into greased casserole, sprinkle on diced potatoes and celery seed. Add about 1 tablespoon vegetable stock. Cover with lid and bake at 400°F/200°C (Gas Mark 6) for 30 minutes. Remove lid and bake for a few minutes longer until top is brown. Serve with nut rissoles and green vegetable — turnip tops or broccoli for preference. Young dandelion leaves would be excellent to serve with this dish in the spring.

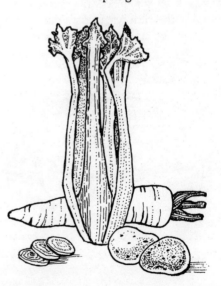

Harvest Pie

4 oz (115g) chestnuts, parboiled, skinned and chopped
1 large carrot, thinly sliced
3 medium onions, thinly sliced
1 cooking apple, chopped
2 sticks celery, sliced
1 tablespoon vegetable oil
2 tomatoes, sliced
1 teaspoon yeast extract, dissolved in a little water
6 oz (170g) short-crust pastry
(see page 111)

1. Lightly fry all ingredients except tomatoes. Place in pie dish with slices of tomato on top.

2. Add yeast extract and cover with pastry. Bake for 30 minutes at 400°F/200°C (Gas Mark 6).

Chestnuts, unlike all other nuts, are not a good source of protein. Therefore, it is advisable to ensure adequate protein by serving this dish with a soya gravy, or have nuts in or with the dessert.

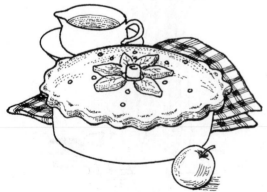

Alankhaan Curry (Madras Style)

1 oz (30g) white fat
2 tablespoons curry powder (mild or full strength according to taste)
1 bay leaf
3 cloves
1 tablespoon lime or lemon juice
Rind of 1 lemon, grated
¼ eating apple, chopped
½ teaspoon sea salt
3-4 tablespoons water
½ oz (15g) coconut or coconut milk made with 1 teaspoon coconut cream dissolved in water
1 teaspoon tomato chutney or ketchup
A little fresh ginger (optional)
1 large onion
1 crushed garlic clove (optional)
½ oz (15g) sultanas
1 tablespoon Barbados sugar

1. Heat the fat in a heavy pan. Stir in the curry powder and other spices for a minute or two. *Keep heat low.*

2. Add other ingredients while continuing to stir over low heat for 10-15 minutes. Taste and add seasoning if necessary. Stir into this sauce whatever is to be curried. Any vegetable would be suitable, also nuts or chestnuts if desired.

3. Cover and leave the flavours to steep for about 30 minutes, keeping hot, but do not allow to boil.

Potato Pie

Mashed potato, seasoned with garlic salt
Sliced onions and tomatoes, fried

1. Place half the mashed potato in a greased pie dish, cover with the tomato and onion mixture and top with the rest of the potato.

2. Reheat in the oven or brown under the grill for a few minutes. Serve with nut rissoles or savoury lentils.

Onion and Chestnut Roast

1 lb (455g) chestnuts, skinned
3 large onions
2 oz (55g) vegan margarine or vegetable oil
2-4 oz (55-115g) wholemeal breadcrumbs
1 dessertspoon yeast extract
Seasoning

1. Cook skinned chestnuts in just sufficient water until almost tender.

2. Chop the onions and cook in the margarine for 5-10 minutes.

3. Add the cooked chestnuts and remaining ingredients and place in a greased baking dish. Bake at 325°F/170°C (Gas Mark 3) for 30-40 minutes.

Chestnut Savoury Crunch

¾ lb (340g) chestnuts
½ lb (225g) onion rings cut into rings
Vegetable oil for frying
A good pinch of sage
½ lb (225g) tomatoes, cut into thick slices
1 oz (30g) vegan margarine
3 oz (85g) fresh wholemeal breadcrumbs

1. Cook skinned chestnuts in a very little water for about 15 minutes. They should not be soft.

2. Fry onion rings in the oil until golden.

3. Place a layer of onions in a greased oven-proof dish and sprinkle on the sage. Cover with chestnuts, then add the tomatoes.

4. Heat the margarine in a pan (use any oil left from the onions for this) and toss the crumbs in this for a few seconds. Sprinkle the crumbs on top and bake in a moderate oven 350°F/180°C (Gas Mark 4) for 20 minutes. If necessary, crisp the top under the grill for a couple of minutes.

Onion and Chestnut Pie

1 lb (455g) chestnuts
1 lb (455g) onions
2 fl oz (60ml) vegetable oil for frying
2½ oz (70g) wholemeal breadcrumbs
1 teaspoon yeast extract
Seasoning
Nut pastry (see page 110)

1. Skin the chestnuts and cook in just sufficient water until tender, not soft.

2. Chop the onions and cook in the oil for 10 minutes.

3. Add the cooked chestnuts and remaining ingredients and place in a greased baking dish.

4. Cover wih nut pastry and bake at 400°F/200°C (Gas Mark 6) for 25-30 minutes. Serve with gravy, a green vegetable and roast potatoes.

Vegetable Roast

Equal quantities of lightly fried onion, carrot and mushroom. 1 teaspoon yeast extract dissolved in a little water. Sufficient mashed potato to cover. Put the fried vegetables into a greased ovenproof dish, pour over yeast extract and cover with potato. Bake at 350°F/180°C (Gas Mark 4) for 30 minutes. Serve with a nut or lentil dish, braised celery and tomatoes.

Edith's Potato Pie

Equal quantities of sliced apple, thinly sliced potatoes and fried onion rings. Seasoning. Put the vegetables into a greased pie dish in layers; potato, onion, apple. Repeat this in this order until the dish is full, finishing with potato slices. Pour over ¼ pint (140ml) vegetable stock and cover wih a greased paper. Bake at 350°F/180°C (Gas Mark 4) for 30 minutes, then uncover and brush with a little oil and brown at 375°F/190°C (Gas Mark 5) for a further 15 minutes. Serve with a nut or lentil dish.

Peach Curry

1lb (455g) tinned peaches, unsweetened
1½ lbs (680g) cooking apples, chopped
1 small onion, chopped
3 tablespoons vegetable oil
1 teaspoon yeast extract
1 pint (570ml) hot water
1 tablespoon curry powder
1 rounded dessertspoon wholemeal flour
Grated rind and juice of ½ lemon
1 oz (30g) ground almonds
2 bananas
1 dessertspoon coconut
Grapes

1. Drain juice from tin of peaches. Gently simmer apples in the juice in a covered pan until almost tender.

2. Lightly fry onion in the oil for a few minutes — do not brown.

3. Dissolve yeast extract in hot water.

4. Mix curry powder and flour together in a basin. Add one teaspoon of flour and curry mixture to pan containing onion and stir in adding small quantity of the water. Continue to do this until you have used it all.

5. Then add lemon rind and juice and almonds. Cook gently until the mixture is thick and creamy.

6. Stir in the cooked apples, peaches and lastly the bananas. Keep stirring gently while reheating the mixture.

7. Just before serving sprinkle top with coconut and grapes.

STUFFED AUBERGINES

3 oz (85g) wholemeal bread
1 small teaspoon yeast extract dissolved in hot water
1 small teaspoon sage
Pinch of sea salt
2 oz (55g) milled walnuts
1 small onion, chopped
1 aubergine

1. Crumble bread and soak in the liquid, adding sage and salt. Fork well and add other ingredients.

2. Remove centre of aubergine and retain this for soup. Stuff with the nut mixture and bake for about 45 minutes in a moderately hot oven, 400°F/200°C (Gas Mark 6).

CAULIFLOWER PIE

1 lightly cooked cauliflower
1 1/2 oz (45g) oil
1 large onion, coarsely grated
4 oz (115g) wholemeal breadcrumbs
Heaped tablespoon finely chopped parsley or teaspoon of mixed herbs
Grated rind of a lemon

1. Chop the cauliflower a little and put into a greased dish.

2. Melt the fat in the pan, add the onion and fry for a few minutes.

3. Stir in the breadcrumbs, the parsley and the lemon rind.

4. Spread this mixture over the cauliflower, press down well, and bake for about 30 minutes in a hot oven, 425°F/220°C (Gas Mark 7).

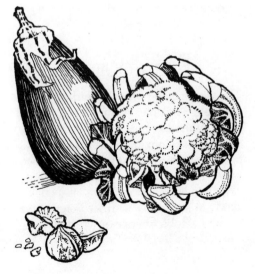

CHESTNUT SAVOURY

1 lb (455g) chestnuts
Just less than ½ lb (225g) onions
2 tablespoons vegetable oil
½ lb (225g) tomatoes
½ oz (15g) wholemeal flour
Seasoning

1. Skin chestnuts (see page 67).

2. Peel, chop and lightly brown onions in fat or oil.

3. Scald, skin and slice the tomatoes. Add enough boiling water to cover and simmer all together until the chestnuts are cooked. Then thicken with flour and season.

4. Serve with a dark green vegetable. This makes 2-3 servings. If there is any that is unused it may be covered with mashed potato or shortcrust pastry for a later meal.

RATATOUILLE

This dish may be varied according to the vegetables available. First fry a large onion in oil. When soft but not brown, add any of the following: marrow or courgettes, cucumber, green or red pepper, tomatoes, aubergine, etc. Season. Add a sprinkle of herbs, if liked. Cover tightly and cook slowly in a casserole without water. Serve with brown rice or wheat.

APPLE AND POTATO PIE

Equal quantities of raw apple, potato and onion, all sliced.

Oil a pie dish and cover bottom with a layer of thin potato slices, sprinkle with celery salt and cover with a layer of thinly sliced onion. Then add a layer of apple, sliced less thinly. Repeat until dish is full, finishing with potato. Add ½ pint (285ml) of vegetable stock and cover with a greased paper on a lid. Cook at 350°F/180°C (Gas Mark 4) for 30 minutes, remove cover and continue cooking at 375°F/190°C (Gas Mark 5) for about 15 minutes. If a casserole is used, allow an extra 15 minutes cooking time.

PARSNIP CRISPIE

Small carrot, chopped
Small parsnip, chopped
Thick white sauce
Small beetroot, cooked and diced
Handful chopped parsley
Seasoning
Curry powder (optional)
Crushed oats

1. Cook carrot and parsnip lightly.

2. Make white sauce and stir in beetroot, parsley, carrot and seasoning.

3. Put into two individual oven-proof dishes, mash parsnip and spread on top.

4. Sprinkle oats over to form the crust and bake in a fairly hot oven at 375°F/190°C (Gas Mark 5) to crisp the topping. Serve with green vegetable and follow with a dish of assorted nuts or a nutty fruit salad.

Baked Beets
(Serves 4)

Three medium sized young beetroots —
raw. Dice into small cubes including skin.
Place in oiled casserole with 2 tablespoons
of water or stock. Bake in oven at
400°F/200° (Gas Mark 6), for 1¼ -1½
hours. Crush 2 oz (55g) roasted cashews
with rolling pin and mix with 2 oz (55g)
finely chopped onions, 1 heaped teaspoon
of chopped fresh mint and 2 tablespoons
vegetable oil. Stir into cooked beets and
serve.

Cornish Pasties

Pease pudding (large or small can)
Equal quantities of left-over vegetable cut
up small
Sprinkling of herbs if desired, fresh if
possible
Short-crust pastry (see page 111)

Roll out wholemeal pastry, cut into saucer
size rounds, cover half generously with the
mixture, damp edges and fold over. Bake
for half an hour at 400°F/200°C (Gas
Mark 6). Serve hot or cold. Excellent for
packed lunches.

Pizza

For the dough:
14 oz (395g) wholemeal flour
1 teaspoon sea salt
½ pint (285ml) warm water
¼ oz (7g) dried yeast
2 tablespoons vegetable oil

Mix, cover and leave in warm place for
1½ -2 hours.

For the topping:
12-14 oz (340-395g) tomatoes, chopped
2 cloves
1 clove garlic
1 teaspoon basil
10 oz (285g) cooked tvp or tin of soya
beans
1 teaspoon marjoram
½ teaspoon sea salt

Heat oven to 425°F/220°C (Gas mark 7).
Peel and finely chop garlic. Add herbs, oil
and tvp meat (or beans). Stir down the
dough and divide into four. Press into
circles on oiled baking sheet; brush with
oil and bake for 10 minutes. Remove from
oven, turn over and cover with topping.
Then return to oven for another 10-15
minutes. This can also be cooked on a
hotplate or in a heavy frying pan when
the oven is not required for anything else.

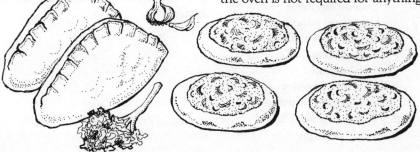

Individual 'Crisp and Nutties'

These dishes cut cooking to a minimum, use very little water, and retain some of the crisp, chewy texture of the vegetables —and more of the natural flavour.

For this method of cooking foods in their own juice, the vegetables are finely sliced or shredded, and served in individual dishes. Wash and prepare any vegetables — (say carrots, celery, onion) by slicing, grating or shredding — and braise in a little oil for 8-10 minutes according to the vegetables being used. Add a few drops of soy sauce if desired and transfer to small dishes. Prepare a thick white sauce, and spread this over so as to cover the vegetables completely. Sprinkle over some millet flakes and crisp under the grill.

Variation:

The covering could be soya 'cheese' or any kind of vegetable which is capable of being pulped in the liquidizer, with a sprinkling of herbs and muesli base.

Onion Tart

Vegetable oil for frying
1 small onion
1 medium carrot
1 medium potato
Small section of cabbage
1 large tomato
Soya sauce
Handful of parsley
2 oz (55g) ground nuts
Pastry flan case, baked 'blind'

1. Lightly fry in the oil the chopped onion, carrot, potato, cabbage and any other vegetables used, except tomato, using a covered pan.

2. After only a few minutes add a good shake of soya sauce and strain off any remaining oil or vegetable juice.

3. Cool, then fill flan case, top with sliced tomato and pop into hot oven 425°F/220°C (Gas Mark 7) for 10 minutes.

Thermos Cookery

Rinse a wide-necked vacuum flask with boiling water, half fill with washed brown rice and other grain. Top with boiling water and leave overnight.

For Vegetables

Bring diced vegetables to the boil, add *Barmene* or other flavouring if liked, and seal in flask. This takes only 3-4 hours to cook.

For Soup

Soup can also be cooked in this way. After rinsing vacuum flask with boiling water shred or liquidize vegetables, add boiling stock or water, salt and a yeast extract such as *Barmene* and leave overnight. Press through a sieve and stir in a generous amount of wheatgerm or bran. Soya sauce can be used in place of salt or yeast extract for variety. Add just before serving.

SMALL SAVOURIES

To add variety and extra nourishment to nut roasts or savoury dishes, replace some of the breadcrumbs (or flour) with muesli base, soya meal or flakes, or millet flakes. When making patties or rissoles it is advisable to whiz the cereals in the blender for a few seconds. This gives a smoother blend and makes for easier moulding.

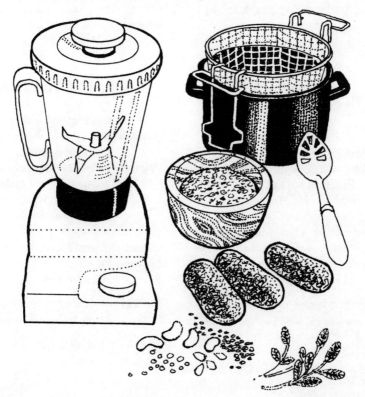

Raw Nut Rissoles

2 oz (55g) ground hazelnuts or Brazils
3 oz (85g) ground cashews
Approx. 1 teaspoon vegetable oil
½ teaspoon dried basil

Mix well together and pound until ingredients adhere. Mould into small balls and roll in any crushed cereal.

For train journeys or school lunches add to the lunchbox some celery, an orange, and a date and banana sandwich for full nutritional value.

These mixtures can be increased in bulk —and made more economical — if a few fresh breadcrumbs and vegetable oil are added.

Pancake or Fritter Mixture

12 fl oz (340ml) water
4½ oz (128g) 81% plain flour
2 rounded tablespoons soya flour
Pinch of sea salt
Vegetable oil for frying.

1. Put water into blender, switch on and add dry ingredients and oil gradually, whiz for about one minute. Leave in a cool place overnight.

2. Beat again just before using. If required for fritters use only 8 fl oz (228ml) water.

Raw Peanut Savouries

4 oz (115g) ground cashew nuts
1 oz (30g) peanut butter
1 teaspoon fresh thyme leaves (or less if dried must be used)
½ oz (15g) grated onion — no more
1 tablespoon lemon juice
1 shredded wheat biscuit

1. Pound together all but the biscuit until ingredients bind.

2. Crumble the shredded wheat biscuit and add to the other ingredients.

3. Form into rissoles and serve with salad, cooked vegetables or use in packed lunches.

Lentil Fritters

4 oz (115g) red lentils
1 rounded tablespoon chopped onion
1 teaspoon herbs
A good ½ pint (285ml) cold water
1 level teaspoon yeast extract
1½ oz (43g) fresh wholemeal breadcrumbs

1. Simmer the lentils, onion and herbs in the water for 15-20 minutes until the lentils are softened.

2. Add yeast extract, then enough breadcrumbs to make a firm mixture.

3. Form into small fritters and coat in flour. Fry in oil until brown on both sides.

Note: This mixture is easier to form into fritters if left to cool first. Should the mixture be too moist, add a little flour.

SOYA FRITTERS

3 heaped tablespoons soya flour
3 heaped tablespoons 100% wholemeal flour
3 heaped tablespoons 81% plain flour
1 teaspoon sage
1 teaspoon yeast extract
1/4 teaspoon sea salt
Cold water to make a fairly thick batter

Beat all ingredients together thoroughly, then allow to stand for 30 minutes. Beat again and fry quickly in very hot oil.

ALAN'S POTATO CAKES

1/2 lb (225g) cooked potatoes
1 large tin bought paté
1 oz (30g) vegan margarine
2 oz (55g) fresh wholemeal breadcrumbs
1 oz (30g) 81% wholemeal flour
Vegetable oil for frying

1. Skin the cooked potatoes while hot and beat in the paté, margarine and breadcrumbs.

2. Add the flour and form into small flat cakes.

3. Shallow fry in oil, lightly, on both sides. If herbs or seasoning are used this should be added sparingly or the delicate flavour of the paté will be lost.

PEASE PUDDING FRITTERS

1 large can pease pudding
2 oz (55g) fine wholemeal breadcrumbs
Chopped chives
1 teaspoon sage
1 teaspoon marjoram

Mix all ingredients thoroughly, form into rissoles, roll in flour and fry in vegetable oil.

ALMOND RISSOLES

1½ tablespoons ground almonds
2 tablespoons breadcrumbs
Pinch of lemon thyme
Pinch of salt and pepper
Pulp of 1 tomato
1 teaspoon grated onion
1 crispbread biscuit

Mix all ingredients but the biscuit together — form into rissoles or rolls, and press in one crushed crispbread biscuit — leave for 2 or 3 hours to set. Sage can be used instead of thyme, and apple sauce or grated apple served with salad if liked.

Paté Savoury

2 tablespoons ground cashews
2 tablespoons ground Brazils
1 oz (30g) vegan margarine
½ teaspoon yeast extract — or rather less
Enough bought paté to flavour and help to
bind (1½ to 2 oz/45-55g)

1. Pound well together, adding paté as necessary.

2. Form into neat shapes and serve with salad. These savouries are excellent for packed lunches and ensure protein in a snack meal.

Lentil Cutlets

4 oz (115g) red lentils
6 oz (170g) potatoes
2 medium onions
2 teaspoons soya flour
1 teaspoon fresh sage or thyme (or ½
teaspoon dried herbs)
1 level teaspoon agar-agar
Seasoning

Coating Batter:
1 tablespoon soya flour
1 tablespooon wholewheat flour
1 tablespoon 81% wholemeal flour
Salt

1. Mix the batter ingredients with water to make a stiff batter and beat well. Allow to stand for at least ½ hour before using.

2. Beat again and use for coating. (This batter can be used for pancakes if a little extra water is added.)

3. Simmer lentils in just over ½ pint (285ml) water or vegetable stock for 20 minutes. Strain, allow to dry and press through sieve (or blend for a few seconds).

4. Cook and mash potato.

5. Chop onions finely and cook in oil for 5 minutes. Season and mix all together thoroughly.

6. Shape into rissoles, dip in coating batter and fry just enough to crisp the batter.

Vegan Sausages

3 oz (85g) tvp mince
½ pint (285ml) brown stock paste
Seasoning
1 oz (30g) wholemeal breadcrumbs
2 tablespoons wholemeal flour
Vegetable oil for mixing and cooking

1. Put mince in blender or grinder to make it finer, then soak in hot stock to soften.

2. Mix a generous amount of seasoning with crumbs and flour. Add to strained mince and mix well, adding oil as necessary.

3. Form into sausage shapes and fry in hot oil, turning frequently. Alternatively brush with oil and grill, or bake in hot oven, 425°F/220°C (Gas Mark 7).

4. Meanwhile make an onion sauce by browning 2 chopped onions in a little hot oil. Add 1 tablespoon flour and cook, stirring, for 5 minutes.

5. Add, gradually ½ pint (285ml) stock mixed with 1 teaspoon bought gravy powder and continue to stir as it cooks and thickens. Serve all with grilled tomatoes and creamed potatoes.

Raw Nut Savoury Rissoles

4 shredded wheat biscuits
5 oz (140g) milled cashews
3 oz (85g) brazil nuts
3 dessertspoons grated carrot
1 teaspoon yeast extract
Tomato juice
1 teaspoon basil

1. Crumble the shredded wheat biscuits, mix with nuts and carrots.

2. Dissolve yeast extract in a little tomato juice and add basil.

3. Add to other ingredients with sufficient extra tomato juice to moisten and bind.

4. Form into balls and serve on green salad. Garnish top of rissoles with chervil or parsley leaves.
Add an apple, a few raisins and a bought paté and cucumber sandwich for a satisfying and adequate packed lunch.

Soya Burgers

½ pint (285ml) stock
2 oz (55g) tvp mince
2 oz (55g) rolled oats
1 teaspoon tomato purée
1 onion (minced)
2 tablespoons wholemeal flour
2 tablespoons vegetable oil
A pinch of mixed herbs and seasoning

1. Dissolve stock powder (if used) in water, add mince, oats, tomato purée, onions, herbs and seasoning.

2. Allow to stand for 5 minutes then add the flour and vegetable oil.

3. Leave for a further 10 minutes and form into flat rissoles (or use a burger press).

4. Cook in hot oil for 5 minutes each side and slide into a wholemeal roll for immediate consumption. Very popular with most children. Alternatively serve with a brown gravy and vegetables.

Individual Mushroom Savouries

4 oz (115g) chopped onions
Vegetable oil for frying
4 oz (115g) mushrooms, chopped
2 teaspoons wholemeal flour
1 teaspoon soya flour
4-5 oz (115-140g) mashed potato
2 oz (55g) wholemeal breadcrumbs
1 handful chopped parsley (optional)
2 teaspoons yeast extract
1 heaped tablespoon millet flakes or other cereal

1. Fry onions light brown in oil, add mushrooms and cook a further few minutes.

2. Mix the flour and soya flour to a paste with a little cold water or stock and stir into vegetables. Allow to boil gently while stirring for a couple of minutes.

3. Add potato, breadcrumbs, parsley and yeast extract. Mix well.

4. Turn into three individual fireproof dishes, sprinkle with cereal flakes and put under the grill to brown and crisp the 'crust'. Serve with any green vegetable, cooked or raw.

Toast Snacks

Baked beans on toast are an excellent source of high quality protein but the quick toast meal does not have to begin and end with beans, tomatoes or mushrooms. Try grated onion with skinned and mashed tomato and sufficient ground cashews to make a creamy toast topping, or mashed avocado mixed with pulped tomato and a drop of lemon juice. Or mix lightly cooked mushrooms with paté, or lightly fried aubergines with mashed potato. Various left-overs can be used in this way.

Carrot Cutlets

6 oz (170g) carrots, washed, scraped and sliced thinly
1 tablespoon vegetable oil for frying
3 tablespoons water (approx)
Seasoning
1 oz (30g) wholemeal flour
1 oz (30g) vegan margarine
¼ pint (140ml) water
2 oz (55g) chopped almonds
2 oz (55g) breadcrumbs
Oatmeal, for coating.

1. Place carrots, oil, water and seasoning in saucepan, bring to the boil and simmer until carrots are tender. Press through sieve (or liquidize).

2. To make a roux, melt the margarine in a pan, then stir well while gradually adding flour to melted margarine. Cook for a couple of minutes before slowly adding the water, still stirring. Cook and stir for a further 3 or 4 minutes.

3. Add to this the chopped almonds, breadcrumbs and seasoning to taste. Stir in carrot mixture and allow to cool.

4. Shape into cutlets, coat with fine oatmeal and fry in hot oil. Serve hot or serve cold with salad.

Unfried Nut Balls

½ teaspoon yeast extract
Hot water to mix
4 oz (115g) fresh wholemeal breadcrumbs
½ lb (225g) ground mixed nuts
1 tablespoon chopped fresh parsley

1. Dissolve the yeast extract in about 4 tablespoons of the hot water. Add the breadcrumbs and about 6 oz (170g) of the nuts.

2. Add parsley, mix well and form into balls.

3. Roll in the remainder of the nuts. As these contain fresh parsley they should be used fairly soon after making. Very handy for lunch boxes or as party snacks.

Parsnip Snacks

2 oz (55g) grated parsnip
2 oz (55g) ground mixed nuts
Vegetable oil
Pinch of salt
1 oz (30g) fresh wholemeal breadcrumbs
Pinch of dried herbs

Pound all together with a little oil until the mixture can be formed into shapes. These can be served with salad without cooking or, if preferred, dipped in a coating batter (see page 80) and lightly fried.

Nuts can usually be bought ready ground from a health food shop or good grocer. However, they will be fresher and cost less if they can be ground at home. An electric blender will do this very well.

To Prepare Brown Rice for Savoury Dishes

Wash 1 tablespoon rice. Add enough water to make up to ½ pint (285ml). Boil for 10 minutes, then reduce heat so that rice is kept just below boiling for approximately half an hour, keeping lid on. Use in any recipe calling for cooked brown rice.

Hints

Tartex Pâté can be used in many ways other than in sandwiches or on toast. Add a little to mashed potatoes, for instance.

From time to time I have tested a recommended cooked rissole mixture which has disintegrated immediately on being introduced to the hot oil.

If this ever happens to you, the balance of the mixture can be used if a little extra ground cashews or breadcrumbs are added to the mixture then dipped in batter before being quickly fried.

Savoury Sauces, Stuffings and Spreads

Sage and Onion Stuffing

½ lb (225g) onions
Vegetable oil for cooking
2 oz (55g) vegan margarine
1 teaspoon chopped sage
Seasoning
2 oz (55g) wholemeal breadcrumbs
Gravy or wholemeal sauce

Chop onions finely, fry until golden brown, add margarine, sage, seasoning and breadcrumbs; bind with gravy or sauce.

Parsley Stuffing

4 oz (115g) wholemeal breadcrumbs
1 oz (30g) vegan margarine (grated)
1 teaspoon thyme
2 tablespoons chopped parsley
Grated rind of ½ lemon
Seasoning
Wholemeal sauce

Mix all dry ingredients together, bind with a little wholemeal sauce.

Chestnut Stuffing II

¾ lb (340g) chestnuts
1 onion, chopped and lightly fried
2 oz (55g) wholemeal breadcrumbs
Seasoning

1. Place chestnuts in a saucepan with cold water, bring to the boil, peel. Cook in ½ pint (285ml) water, strain and mash.

2. Add fried onion, breadcrumbs and seasoning and mix to stiff consistency.

Chestnut Balls

To each 5 oz (140g) of cooked, sieved chestnuts (the approximate result of ½ lb/225g) add a little salt and about 1 oz (30g) vegan margarine and blend well. Roll into quite small balls. If liked roll in any finely chopped fresh herbs. Serve with green salad or around a nut roast.

Savoury Sauces

Béchamel (White Sauce De Luxe)

1 slice onion
1 sprig of parsley
1 sprig of thyme
1 bay leaf (small)
½ pint (285ml) hot vegetable stock
1½ oz (45g) vegan margarine
1 oz (30g) wholemeal flour
Sea salt
Pinch of ground mace or grated nutmeg

1. Add the onion, parsley, thyme and bay leaf to the hot stock in pan.

2. Bring to the boil. Strain. Set aside.

3. In another pan melt the margarine and add the flour and salt. Cook over low heat for 1-2 minutes. Continue stirring while slowly adding strained liquid.

4. Cook gently while stirring for a few minutes. Add mace to taste, cover and keep warm.

Parsley Sauce

To vary white sauce, leave out mace, thyme and bay leaf and add a good handful of fresh, chopped parsley, when cooked.

Apple and Onion Sauce

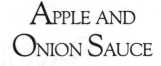

2 large cooking apples
3 medium-sized onions, peeled
1 oz (30g) vegan margarine
2 teaspoons Barbados sugar
Seasoning

1. Slice apples and chop onions. Put into pan with margarine, sugar and seasoning.

2. Cook gently with lid on until soft, or in casserole if oven is in use.

Quick Leek Sauce

Well wash and cut up 1 large or 2 small leeks. Steam until soft for 10-15 minutes. Strain but keep the stock. In another pan make a roux with 1 oz (30g) margarine or oil, 1 oz (30g) wholemeal flour and seasoning. Gradually add the stock while stirring to a creamy consistency, adding more water if necessary. Stir in leeks and serve with any hot savoury dish.

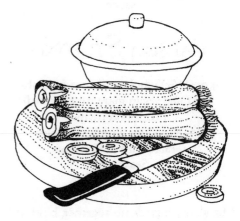

PASTES AND SPREADS

WALNUT PASTE

1 small onion, chopped finely
1 oz (30g) vegan margarine
4 oz (115g) tomatoes
2 oz (55g) milled walnuts
2 oz (55g) wholemeal breadcrumbs
Seasoning

1. Fry onion in margarine then add tomatoes, skinned and chopped. Lastly add walnuts, breadcrumbs and seasoning.

2. Mix well together, lightly. When cold it is ready for use.

LENTIL PASTE

1 small onion, chopped finely
1 oz (30g) vegan margarine
¼ teaspoon powdered sage
4 oz (115g) lentils
½ pint (285ml) vegetable stock
2 oz (55g) wholemeal breadcrumbs
Celery salt
Seasoning

1. Braise onion with margarine in saucepan, add powdered sage, lentils and stock. Cook gently, stirring frequently.

2. When cooked, pass through sieve, add breadcrumbs and seasoning, mix well. When cold it is ready for use.

TOMATO AND PARSLEY SAUCE

½ lb (225g) onion
½ oz (15g) vegan margarine
½ lb (225g) tomatoes
½ oz (15g) wholemeal breadcrumbs
1 salt-spoon grated horseradish
1 tablespoon chopped parsley
Seasoning

1. Chop onion finely, fry golden brown in the margarine.

2. Peel and chop tomatoes, and add to onions.

3. When cooked add all other ingredients, mix well. When cold it is ready for use, or can be made into small balls and served on a plate, garnished with parsley.

SAVOURY SPREAD

Cream peanut butter with wooden spoon and mix in any finely chopped herbs in season and a small quantity of yeast extract. Alternatively, a little grated raw onion or finely chopped mushroom can be used. This spread should be made as required as it will not keep for more than a few hours due to the fresh herbs. Excellent for protein sandwiches in a lunch box.

Celery Spread

Mix minced celery (say three centre stalks) with about eight grated Brazil nuts. Pound well together and spread on bread or rolls with margarine or home-made cream cheese.

Parsley Butter

Blend one tablespoon of chopped parsley into four ounces of vegan margarine or nut butter. Add half a teaspoon of paprika. Alternative flavours are chives, apple mint, dill, etc. All herbs must be fresh for this purpose.

Gravies

Quick Brown Gravy

**1 oz (30g) vegan margarine
1 teaspoon yeast extract
½ oz (15g) wholemeal flour
1 teaspoon gravy browning
½ pt (285ml) vegetable stock
A pinch of garlic powder or other seasoning if required**

1. Warm oil or margarine, stir in yeast extract and remove from heat. Blend in the flour and mix well.

2. Add the gravy mix to the stock and gradually stir this into the mixture over a low heat.

3. Bring to the boil while stirring and simmer for a minute or two. Taste for seasoning.

Rich Gravy

After frying vegetables such as tomatoes, onions or aubergines in oil, add a good teaspoon of wholemeal flour to the remaining oil in the pan, stir while gently cooking for a minute or so, add water or stock slowly until suitable consistency, add a few drops of soya sauce to flavour, and strain. If more colour is desired, use half flour and half commercial gravy mix.

Desserts and Ice Cream

Sugarless Apricot Sweet

2 oz (55g) apricots (soaked to soften)
1 teaspoon agar-agar

Liquidize fruit and water and make up to ½ pint (285ml) if necessary. Heat gently in pan and sprinkle in agar-agar while stirring. Simmer, stirring for 2 minutes. Leave to cool and serve with chopped nuts and vegan cream (see page 97).

Apple Vinny

3 apples
1 oz (30g) fruit sugar
1 tablespoon orange juice
1-2oz (30-55g) vegan margarine
2 slices of wholemeal bread (approx)

1. Wash and chop apples. Cook together with sugar and orange juice (a small quantity of water may be necessary with some apples).

2. Melt margarine in saucepan. Cut bread into fingers, then coat with melted margarine; turn so that both sides are coated.

3. Put stewed apple into shallow oven-proof dish, cover with the bread and sprinkle over a little sugar. Put under the grill for a few minutes to brown.

No-Egg Pancakes

12 fl oz (340ml) water
4½ oz (128g) wholemeal flour
3 rounded tablespoons soya flour
Pinch sea salt
Vegetable oil for frying

1. Pour water into blender, switch on and add dry ingredients gradually. Whiz for about 1 minute. Leave in cool place for at least 1 hour. (Can be left in refrigerator overnight.)

2. Beat again just before using. (If required for fritters use only 8 fl oz (228ml) water.)

3. Fry on both sides in very lightly oiled pan and serve while hot with lemon juice and fruit sugar or syrup.

Fruit Medley

½ lb (225g) stoned dates
2 bananas
2 oz (55g) chopped nuts
2 oz (55g) seedless raisins (soaked for 15 minutes)
Grated rind and juice of an orange

1. Mix all ingredients well together, adding enough orange juice to make the mixture stiff. Press into basin.

2. When required turn out and serve with soya milk.

Christmas Pudding

½ lb (225g) stoned raisins
½ lb (225g) seedless raisins
½ lb (225g) currants
½ lb (225g) sultanas
4 oz (115g) mixed peel
½ lb (225g) Barbados sugar
¼ teaspoon grated nutmeg
½ teaspoon pudding spice
6 oz (170g) wholemeal breadcrumbs
2 oz (55g) chopped almonds
½ lb (225g) vegetable suet
2 oz (55g) wholemeal flour
½ pint (285ml) orange juice

1. Put washed and dried fruit into a large bowl with chopped peel, sugar, spices, breadcrumbs, nuts, fat and flour.

2. Stir in enough orange juice to moisten, and allow to stand overnight.

3. Next day, if necessary, add a little extra moisture — juice or spirits as desired — and pack tightly into a greased basin, cover with greased greaseproof paper or cooking foil and a cloth. Steam for 8 hours.

4. A further good steaming of 2 to 3 hours on the day it is to be served will improve the flavour. Serve with concentrated soya milk, cream or, if preferred, a custard can be made with a vegetable milk.

Mince Pies

For pastry:
2 oz (30g) white fat
2 oz (30g) vegan margarine
½ lb (225g) wholemeal flour
2 oz (30g) fruit sugar
Cold water

1. Rub the fats into the flour, add sugar, mix with just enough cold water to make a soft dough.

2. Roll out thinly and line patty tins.

3. Add mincemeat, cover with pastry and snip the top. Bake at 400°F/200°C (Gas Mark 6) for 25 minutes.

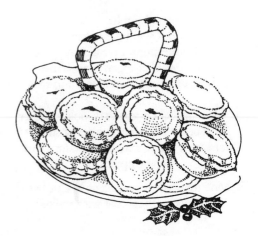

Apricot Flip

**About 16 apricot halves (soaked
overnight)
4 fl oz (115ml) of the juice
1 small tablespoon Barbados sugar or
fruit sugar
2 teaspoons lemon rind finely grated
2 tablespoons lemon juice
2 teaspoons agar-agar
2 tablespoons home-made nut cream
(see page 98)**

1. Press apricots through strainer (or whiz
in blender). Add the juice.

2. Add sugar, lemon rind and juice to the
apricot purée and heat to boiling point.
Remove from heat and sift in agar-agar.

3. When cool, fold in the nut cream and
pour into individual dishes to set.

Dutch Apple Tart

**1 quantity wholemeal pastry
(see page 110)
2 oz (55g) dates
½ lb (225g) grated apple
1 oz (30g) brown sugar
Juice and rind of ½ lemon**

1. Line a sandwich tin with wholemeal
pastry.

2. Chop dates, add grated apples, sugar
and juice and mix well.

3. Fill tin and cover with another round of
thin pastry. Prick to allow steam to escape
and cook in a hot oven at 400°F/200°C
(Gas Mark 6) for 30 minutes.

Orange Flan

**Shortcrust pastry (see page 111)
3 or 4 oranges
1 oz (30g) ground almonds
Peel from 1 lemon
2 oz (55g) fruit sugar
1 oz (30g) cornflour**

1. Make and cook flan case.

2. Fill flan case with sections of oranges
and the almonds.

3. Make a stock with the rinds of oranges
and the lemon and ½ pint (285ml) of
water. Remove rinds, add sugar and mix
cornflour with a little water. Stir together.

4. Cook liquid until clear and when cool
— but not set — pour over oranges in
flan.

Marmalade Pudding

**3 oz (85g) 81% self-raising flour
1 oz (30g) soya flour
1 level teaspoon baking powder
2 oz (55g) vegan margarine
1 tablespoon marmalade in the bottom of a
greased pudding basin**

1. Sift together dry ingredients and rub in
margarine.

2. Mix to a soft dough with the liquid.

3. Turn into a greased basin, cover and
steam for 1 hour. Jam or syrup can be
used instead of marmalade.

Family Slices (Bread Pudding)

Soak stale bread in water for 10-15 minutes. Press out excess water and to each 12 oz (340g) add:
2 oz (55g) brown sugar
3 oz (85g) mixed fruit, including peel
1 oz (30g) vegetable suet
1 heaped teaspoon mixed cake spice

1. Mix all ingredients well.

2. Bake in greased ovenproof dish for about 3 hours at a very low temperature, 225°F/110°C (Gas Mark ¼).

3. When cold, cut into slices and sprinkle with coconut or finely chopped almonds.

Coffee and Walnut Dessert

2 teaspoons agar-agar
1 tablespoon strong decaffeinated coffee
1 pint (570ml) boiling water
2 oz (55g) Barbados sugar
1 good tablespoon nut cream
(see page 98)
2 oz (55g) chopped walnuts

1. Mix the agar-agar and the hot coffee to a smooth paste, add boiling water and sugar and stir well.

2. Then add the nut cream, whisk well, pour into individual dishes and decorate with chopped walnuts. Serve with a vegan cream or undiluted concentrated vegetable milk for a special treat.

Open Apple Tart

½ lb (225g) cooking apples and 1 small eating apple
1 oz (30g) Barbados sugar
2 oz (55g) sultanas
½ lemon
1 quantity wholemeal pastry
(see page 110)

1. Cook the apples except one, add sugar, sultanas, grated rind and juice of lemon and mix well.

2. Line a shallow tin with wholemeal pastry, prick the bottom and cook at 400°F/200°C (Gas Mark 6).

3. When the pastry case is cold, fill with apple mixture and cover with rings of the raw apple. Sprinkle with a little coconut. Serve with a vegan cream or undiluted concentrated vegetable milk. Alternatively, use ½ oz (15g) fruit sugar in place of brown.

Soya Crispie

1 tablespoon wholemeal flour
2 teaspoons soya flour
1 oz (30g) vegan margarine
2 teaspoons Barbados sugar
1 lb (455g) stewed apples, sweetened

1. Sieve flours together and rub in margarine. Add sugar.

2. Sprinkle this mixture over fruit in a shallow ovenproof dish and bake for 30 minutes at 300°F/150°C (Gas Mark 2) or until top is golden colour. Can be seved hot or cold.

CHOCOLATE AND DATE MOULD

4 oz (115g) dates, stoned
¾ pint (425ml) water
1 level tablespoon cocoa
¾ level tablespoon Barbados sugar
1 level teaspoon agar-agar
½ teaspoon vanilla essence

1. Wash and chop dates and simmer in half of the water for about five minutes.

2. Mix cocoa, sugar and agar-agar together and pour on the remaining water. Add to dates and stir well until boiling point is reached.

3. Remove from heat and stir in vanilla essence. Strain before pouring into dishes to cool. Serve with *Delice* or home-made nut cream (see page 98).

MINCEMEAT TART

4 oz (115g) mincemeat
About 6 oz (170g) chopped apple
½ lb (225g) shortcrust pastry

1. Mix the mincemeat and apple.

2. Line a pie plate with half the pastry, fill with the fruit mixture and cover with the rest of the pastry.

3. Bake for 30 minutes at 375°F/190°C (Gas Mark 5). The addition of the apple makes the tart not only juicy but more economical.

SWISS APPLE PUDDING

1 lb (455g) apples (Bramley's are best)
3 or 4 cloves
1 oz (30g) raw cane sugar (or ½ oz/15g fructose if sweet is for diabetic)
4 oz (115g) muesli base
2 oz (55g) vegan margarine

1. Core, slice and gently cook apples with cloves. Drain off any surplus juice, stir in sugar and pour into greased pie dish.

2. Measure muesli base into separate bowl, add softened margarine and stir together.

3. Spread over apples in pie dish and bake for 20 minutes at 350°F/180°C (Gas Mark 4).

APPLE CRUMBLE

1 lb (455g) cooking apples
1 tablespoon Barbados sugar or fruit sugar
2 heaped tablespoons wholemeal flour
1 heaped tablespoon soya flour
2 oz (55g) vegan margarine

1. Slice peeled apples into greased casserole dish and sprinkle sugar over.

2. Mix together the remaining dry ingredients and rub in the margarine. Sprinkle over the apple and bake in moderate oven at 350°F/180°C (Gas Mark 4) for 20 minutes or until brown.

Bread and Butter Pudding

2 large slices of wholemeal bread, spread
with vegan margarine
1 tablespoon raw cane sugar
2 oz (55g) mixed dried fruit
Grated rind of an orange
½ pint (285ml) vegetable milk
1 bare teaspoon agar-agar
A few drops vanilla essence
Nutmeg

1. Slice the bread and margarine into neat
pieces to fit the oven dish to be used. Place
a layer in the bottom of the dish,
margarine side down.

2. Sprinkle bread with some of the sugar
and fruit. Repeat, using the rest of the
sugar, fruit and rind, leaving enough of
the bread to cover the top.

3. Warm the milk and dissolve the agar-
agar in it.

4. Add flavouring (if used) and pour over
the bread in the dish. Sprinkle lightly
with nutmeg and put aside for about 30
minutes.

5. Cook in the oven for 25 minutes at
400°F/200C° (Gas Mark 6).

Orange Jelly

2 oranges
2 teaspoons agar-agar
2 teaspoons Barbados sugar
½ pt (285ml) boiling water
2 teaspoons nut cream (see page 98)
Few chopped almonds

1. Wash the oranges and grate the rind of
one of them into a bowl.

2. Mix the juice with the agar-agar adding
the sugar and half of the boiling water.

3. Mix well the rest of the water with the
nut cream (in electric mixer if possible)
and add to the agar-agar mixture and the
grated peel.

4. Pour into a wetted mould (or small
dishes) and decorate with thin slices of
orange and chopped nuts.

Chocolate Flavoured Ice-cream

½ tin carob concentrated soya milk
1 level teaspoon agar-agar
1 tablespoon sugar
1 vanilla pod or 8 drops of vanilla essence

1. Mix agar-agar with sugar and add milk.
Bring *almost* to the boil stirring all the time
over low heat with vanilla pod. If a vanilla
pod is not available add the essence *after
removing from the heat*.

2. Freeze in ice compartment for 1 hour,
take out and beat thoroughly before
returning to freezer for another hour, or
longer, if necessary.

Stuffed Oranges

3 oranges
About 12 dates
2 ripe dessert apples
A few nuts

1. Cut the oranges in half and carefully scoop out the pulp into a basin. Remove the pith, leaving the skins clean.

2. Chop the dates very finely, grate the apples, and mix all with the orange pulp.

3. Pile the mixture back into the cases and top with milled nuts mixed with a little of the orange juice.

Fresh Orange Compote

4-5 oranges according to size
½ lb (225g) Barbados sugar
1 pint (570ml) water
Juice of 2 lemons

1. Wash the oranges, add the grated rind of two oranges to the sugar and water and boil gently without stirring until the syrup is thick. Stir in the strained lemon juice.

2. While the syrup is cooking, remove all white pith from the oranges and cut into ¼-inch (½cm) slices.

3. Lay orange slices in a large shallow dish, pour the hot syrup over them and leave in a cool place until required.

Apple and Date Mousse

1 lb (455g) apples
½ lb (225g) dates
Juice of an orange
1 tablespoon coconut cream

1. Stew the apples until soft.

2. Wash, stone and chop the dates into small pieces and mash well with the apple.

3. Add the orange juice and beat in the nut cream while the mixture is still hot.

4. Pour into dish and leave to cool.

Carob Mould

2 teaspoons agar-agar
1¼ pints (710ml) cold water
2 teaspoons carob flour
1 tablespoon nut cream (see page 98)
2 tablespoons Barbados sugar
A little vanilla essence

1. Mix the agar-agar with ¼ pint (140ml) of cold water.

2. Boil the remaining 1 pint (570ml) of water. Use about half to mix the carob.

3. Mix the nut cream to a smooth milk with the rest of the hot water.

4. Bring the carob liquid to the boil with the agar-agar, stirring all the time. Allow to boil for a minute or two, then stir in sugar, nut cream and essence.

5. Pour into a mould and leave to set.

Lemon and Barley Jelly

1 oz (30g) barley kernels (2 tbs)
1 pint (570ml) water
Juice of 1 lemon
1 inch (2.5cm) cinnamon stick (or pinch of powdered cinnamon)

1. Boil all ingredients together gently for ¾ hour, until it becomes thick and transparent.

2. Strain, sweeten to taste, pour into rinsed mould. Serve with vegan cream, home-made nut cream or undiluted concentrated soya milk.

'Chocolate' Blancmange

1 tin carob concentrated soya milk
6 tablespoons cornflour
½ pint (285ml) water
3 tablespoons sugar

1. Mix 6 tablespoons of the milk with the cornflour into a smooth paste.

2. Put the rest of the milk, the water and the sugar into a pan and bring to the boil.

3. Pour, stirring thoroughly, into the prepared 'paste', return to the saucepan and bring again to the boil, stirring all the time.

4. Pour into dish and allow to cool before placing in fridge.

Junket

½ teaspoon agar-agar
½ pint (285ml) concentrated soya milk
¼ pint (140ml) water
2 teaspoons fruit sugar

1. Dissolve agar-agar in milk and water.

2. Bring to the boil while stirring and simmer for 2 minutes, add sugar.

3. Leave to set. Serve with fresh or stewed fruit.

Fruit Flip

3 large bananas
Half this quantity of any other fresh juicy fruit
2 oz (55g) cashew nuts

1. Liquidize fruit in blender.

2. Then add cashew nuts and switch on again.

3. Remove and chill in individual bowls. Just before serving sprinkle with roughly chopped almonds or Brazil nuts.

Frozen Fruit Nog

Blend in liquidizer 5 oz (140g) frozen strawberries and 2 tablespoons soya milk. Any other frozen fruit may be substituted if desired. Ready to serve immediately.

Banana Ice-Cream

3/4 pint (425ml) soya milk
with 1/4 pint (140ml) water
1/4 pint (140ml) vegetable oil
1/4 pint (140ml) maple syrup
2 bananas

1. Put diluted milk into blender and add oil slowly while running. Add syrup and bananas and whiz again.

2. Pour into dish and place in freezer compartment of refrigerator. To prevent slivers of ice forming in the cream, remove from container when partially frozen and beat again.

3. Return to freezer until quite firm. Serve with blackcurrant juice or other fruit syrup and sprinkle with chopped nuts.

Non-Dairy Cream

4 oz (115g) vegan margarine
1/4 pint (140ml) nut milk (diluted nut cream)
2 teaspoons lemon juice
1 level tablespoon sugar
Few drops vanilla essence

1. Heat margarine and milk in saucepan (do not boil), add lemon juice, sugar, vanilla. Cool quickly in fridge.

2. Emulsify in electric blender or cream machine. Return to fridge until required.

Note: The choice and availability of nut creams is limited. You might prefer to make the Confectioner's Custard overleaf.

Plamil Ice-Cream

1/2 level teaspoon agar-agar
1 tablespoon syrup
7 fl oz (200ml) concentrated soya milk
Vanilla pod

1. Mix agar-agar with syrup and add *Plamil* and vanilla pod. Bring almost to the boil, stirring all the time over low heat. Add 8 drops vanilla essence after taking off the heat if not using vanilla pod.

2. Freeze for 2 hours, beating thoroughly after the first hour to prevent crystal formation. Serve with fruit syrup.

Fruit Mould

Cook 1/2 lb (225g) of blackcurrants or other soft fruit in season in 1/2 pint (285ml) of water with 1 oz (30g) raw cane sugar. Press through sieve. Mix 2 oz (55g) ground rice to a paste with water, pour into boiling fruit juice, stir until thick. Pour into mould. Turn out when set, and serve with nut cream.

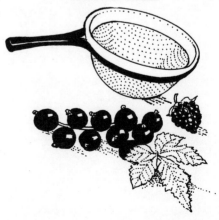

Confectioner's Custard

½ pint (285ml) milk
2 tablespoons cornflour
1-2 oz (30-60g) margarine
1 oz (30g) sugar, pale brown or icing

1. Mix cornflour with the milk and boil until thickened, stirring constantly. Cool completely. To avoid a skin forming, lay a damp film or paper directly onto the custard.

2. Cream the margarine and the sugar together. If you use brown sugar you will finish with a white cream. If you decide to use icing sugar, mix it with a *very* little milk first.

3. Gradually beat the cream into the cold custard. The more you beat, the better it will get. It will thicken more with standing.

Note: The secret of success is to have the custard completely cold, so that there is no risk of the margarine melting, even slightly, which will give a different result.

Home-Made Nut Cream

1 oz (30g) finely ground almonds or Brazils
1 oz (30g) finely ground cashew nuts
¾ oz (20g) vegan margarine (quantities according to the consistency desired)

1. Pound well together until quite smooth, then add a little fresh fruit juice — orange is favourite.

2. If the cream is not immediate use, replace the fruit juice with a few drops of natural vanilla essence.

Carob Flour

Use carob flour to give a chocolate flavour to desserts. It can also be sprinkled on fresh fruit salad at time of serving. Carob flour is nourishing as well as being sweet and flavoursome. Or toss some grated coconut into a little carob flour and use as a topping for any sweet dish.

Bananas, avocados and coconuts are often considered fattening, and avoided for this reason, but they should not add weight if consumed with other compatible (non-animal) foods.

Bread, Cakes and Buns

We derive a good proportion of our protein and other nutrients from bread and the best bread is that which we bake at home. Not only does it give the cook a real sense of satisfaction, but all the family will appreciate the superior flavour of home-made bread. The protein, vitamin B_{12}, calcium and iron value can be raised even more by the addition of soya flour, molasses and concentrated vegetable milk. (See Tiger's Bread, page 102). Try varying the flavour of your bread — and add extra nutrients — by replacing some of the flour with potato, rye or barley flour, wheatgerm, bran, ground nuts or oatmeal.

Try to have everything warm. Grease, flour and warm the tins. In cold weather put the bowl of flour in a warm place for a while. When proving the dough, do not leave it longer than is necessary to raise the loaf to about twice its size after kneading. If left too long, hoping for an even taller loaf, hollows are liable to form under the crust making the finished loaf more difficult to slice neatly. When the loaf slides easily from the tin and sounds 'hollow' when tapped it can be taken from the oven and left to cool on a wire tray.

Fresh yeast is not always easily available, but don't let this deter you from bread-making. Dried yeast works equally well and is always ready for use.

If following a recipe calling for white flour, allow for the fact that wholemeal flour will require a little more water when making bread, pastry, etc.

Home bakers all have their favourite method for bread-making; for example, to get a good crust on brown bread, when cooked turn off heat, remove loaf from tin and replace in oven for a further 10 minutes.

Quick Wholemeal Bread

Try this new quick way of making bread. It really is very simple, and a great time-saver.

This quantity makes 1 loaf or 12 rolls.

1 oz (30g) fresh yeast
1 lb (455g) mixed plain flours, wholemeal and strong white, in any proportion
1 teaspoon salt
½ pint (285ml) water at blood heat*

1. Rub yeast into flour and salt, add all the water and mix to a soft dough. Work to a smooth elastic consistency, dusting the hands with flour if inclined to stick.

2. Place into well-greased (or non-stick) bread tin. Put inside a large polythene bag, loosely tied, and allow to rise to double size.

3. Remove bag. Bake on middle shelf of hot oven, 450°F/230°C (Gas Mark 8) for 35-40 minutes.

*In the absence of a thermometer, the correct temperature can be achieved by adding one part boiling water to two parts cold water.

Baking For One

It is quite easy to make just one small loaf at a time, an added advantage for the person living alone — or the only one in the family with food reform ideas and a palate to match.
For one small loaf you will need:

½ lb wholemeal flour
(or 7 oz/200g wholemeal and 1 oz/30g strong white)
1 teaspoon dried yeast
6-7 fl oz (170-200ml) water at blood heat
½ teaspoon sea salt

1. Light oven, grease and flour bread tin.

2. Put flour and bread tin to warm slightly.

3. Sprinkle the yeast onto the warm water and stir in. Leave in the warm to dissolve thoroughly (10-15 minutes).

4. Add salt to flour. Add yeasty water. Mix well and knead with the hands. This takes about 5 minutes. The dough should be moist enough to handle easily without being sticky. If it is too wet a little extra flour can be sprinkled on and worked in. (It is not possible to give the exact water quantity as flours vary in the amount required to give the same effect. This could be due to the place where the wheat was grown, the weather at the time, or the condition of the soil. Presumably the length of time which has elapsed since it was milled would also have some little effect.)

5. Choose a tin large enough for twice the quantity of bread dough. Form the dough to fit the tin to be used, loosely cover it

with a damp cloth or greaseproof paper and leave in a warm place, out of the draught, to rise. This will take 20-30 minutes.

6. When the dough has risen to about twice its size, put into the pre-heated oven at 450°F/230°C (Gas Mark 8), and bake for 30 minutes.

LONG BREAD ROLLS

1½ lbs (680g) 100% wholemeal flour
1 heaped teaspoon sea salt
1 oz (30g) fresh yeast (or ½ oz/15g dried may be used in accordance with instructions on packet)
About ¾ pint (425ml) of lukewarm water

1. Mix flour and salt.

2. Break down yeast in ¼ pint (140ml) of water.

3. Make depression in flour, pour in yeast and remaining water; stir thoroughly with a large wooden spoon. Then knead for 2 or 3 minutes, using a little more flour if dough is too sticky. Divide dough into six pieces, pull and roll until about 12 inches (30cm) long. Shape nicely (one may indent slantwise with back of knife for decoration).

4. Lay on warmed, greased baking sheets, cover with cloth or polythene and leave to rise 15-20 minutes.

5. Bake for 35-40 minutes at 400°F/200°C (Gas Mark 6).

FRUIT AND NUT LOAF

4 oz (115g) dates (or other dried fruit), roughly chopped
7 fl oz (200ml) soya milk
A bare 3 oz (85g) black treacle
2 oz (55g) vegan margarine (softened)
12 oz (340g) plain wholemeal flour
2½ level teaspoons baking powder
½ teaspoon sea salt
½ level teaspoon bicarbonate of soda
3 oz (85g) Barbados sugar
2 oz (55g) walnuts, roughly chopped ·

1. Warm, grease and flour a bread tin.

2. Wash and dry dates.

3. Warm the milk, treacle and fat together until just melted.

4. Sift dry ingredients together and stir in the sugar.

5. Add the fruit and nuts, stir in the liquid and mix well to a fairly thick, smooth batter.

6. Turn into tin and bake for an hour at 325°F/170°C (Gas Mark 3). Allow to cool partially before turning out onto rack.

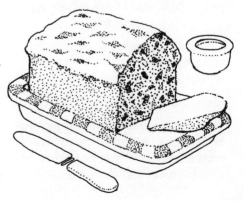

Tiger's Bread

To make one loaf:
13 oz (370g) wholemeal flour
1 teaspoon molasses
2 full teaspoons dried yeast
1 teaspoon sea salt
1 oz (30g) bran
1 oz (30g) soya flour
1 tablespoon ground cashews
12 fl oz (340ml) warm water (101°F/38°C)
2 teaspoons soya flour

1. Heat oven to 450°F/230°C (Gas Mark 8). Grease and flour bread tin.

2. Mix flours and nuts in large bowl.

3. Take 3 fl oz (90ml) of the warm water and sprinkle the yeast onto it. Put this in a warm place to dissolve and froth up (10-20 minutes).

4. Meanwhile, dissolve the molasses and salt in the rest of the water.

5. Make a well in the centre of the flours and pour in the yeast mixture and the molasses water. Mix well with the hands or a wooden spoon. When no dry flour remains, transfer the dough to a wooden board or table, and knead well for a good 5 minutes.

6. Shape the dough, put into warm tin and leave to rise in a warm place until it has almost doubled its bulk.

7. Bake for 30 minutes in centre of oven.

When cooking with yeast nothing must be allowed to get cold, neither should water above blood heat be used as this could 'kill' the yeast.

Small Fruit Cakes

6 oz (170g) wholemeal flour
1 oz (30g) soya flour
1 oz (30g) wheatgerm
4 oz (115g) vegan margarine
2 oz (55g) fruit sugar
4 oz (115g) dried fruit
2 oz (55g) chopped peel
1 heaped teaspoon cake spice (optional)
Rather less than 1 teaspoon bicarbonate of soda
2 oz (55g) coconut
Grated rind and juice of 1 lemon
1 level teaspoon cream of tartar
Water to mix (5-6 fl oz/140-170ml)

1. Sieve flours and wheatgerm together.

2. Cream fat and fruit sugar well.

3. Mix in flours and fruit and all remaining ingredients adding water (or vegetable milk) until just soft enough to beat. Beat briskly for 3 minutes.

4. Fill 24 paper cases or tins and bake for 18 minutes at 375°F/190°C (Gas Mark 5) in centre of oven. For festive touch, decorate with pieces of angelica, walnut or glacé cherries just before baking.

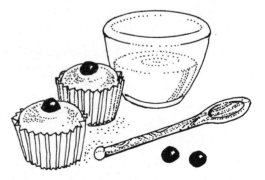

SPONGE SANDWICH

4 oz (115g) white fat
1 heaped tablespoon cane sugar
3 oz (85g) Barbados sugar
½ lb (225g) 81% self-raising flour
1 level teaspoon bicarbonate of soda
Warm water to mix

1. Melt fat, syrup and sugar together and add flour.

2. Dissolve bicarbonate of soda in 5 fl oz (140ml) warm water and add to mixture stirring all the time. Add more water if necessary to make a soft mixture. Beat well.

3. Place in two sandwich tins which have been previously warmed, greased and floured. Bake at 400°F/200°C (Gas Mark 6) for 20 minutes.

CHOCOLATE BUNS

4 oz (115g) white fat
3 oz (85g) Barbados sugar
1 level teaspoon cream of tartar
Rather less than 1 level teaspoon bicarbonate of soda
2 teaspoons soya flour
7 oz (200g) wholemeal flour
1 oz (30g) carob flour

1. Cream fat and sugar thoroughly.

2. Sift dry ingredients together.

3. Gradually add these to fat mixture, adding a little water if necessary to make a good beating consistency. Beat well.

4. Divide into 24 and bake in centre of oven for 18 minutes at 375°F/190°C (Gas Mark 5).

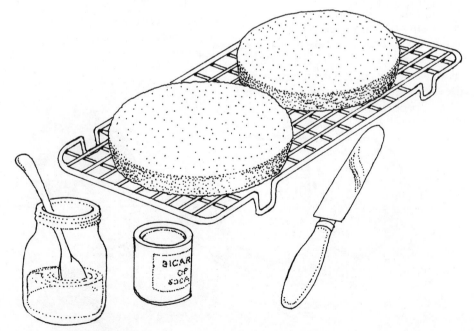

Kathleen's Rich Fruit Cake

¾ lb (340g) currants
½ lb (225g) seedless raisins
¾ lb (340g) sultanas
½ pint (285ml) water
6 tablespoons vegetable oil
1 tablespoon dark treacle
1 teaspoon spice
Lemon and orange rind, finely grated
1 teaspoon arrowroot (optional)
14 oz (395g) self-raising wholemeal flour

1. Wash fruit and add water, oil, treacle, spice, grated rinds, and mix well together.

2. Make arrowroot into a thin cream with 2 tablespoons of water and stir into the mixture.

3. Lightly stir in the flour and mix well.

4. Grease and line a large cake tin, spoon in the cake mixture and bake in the centre of the oven for 3 hours at 225°F/110°C (Gas Mark ¼). After half an hour cover the cake with another piece of greaseproof paper to prevent burning.

Food Reform Cakelets
(Uncooked)

1 tablespoon wheatgerm
2 tablespoons whole rolled oats or muesli base
1 tablespoon Barbados sugar (or 2 rounded teaspoons fruit sugar)
2 tablespoons nut butter or vegan margarine
Some lemon juice and ground almonds or cashews

1. Mix the dry ingredients and work in the fat.

2. Add lemon juice until the mixture will hold together.

3. Form into small balls by rolling in the hands and roll in the ground nuts. Put aside in a cool place to set. These are very quick and easy to make and the recipe lends itself to many variations of cereals and flavours. Cocoa or carob flour could be used in place of nuts.

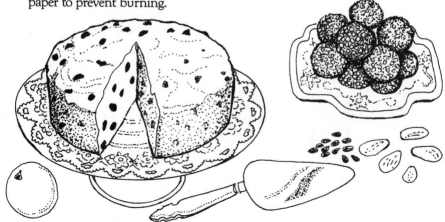

Carob Fairy Cakes

3 fl oz (90ml) vegetable oil
8 fl oz (230ml) water
2 oz (55g) light soft brown sugar
6½ oz (185g) 81% self-raising flour
1 heaped teaspoon baking powder
1½ oz (45g) carob flour

Filling:
2 oz (55g) very fine sugar
A few drops of vanilla essence
2 oz (55g) vegan margarine

1. Stir oil into water and beat lightly into mixed dry ingredients (by hand) for 2 minutes.

2. Bake for 15 minutes at 350°F/180°C (Gas Mark 4).

3. For the filling, cream all ingredients together. When cakes are cold, remove the tops with a sharp knife and put a little of the butter icing under the 'lid' of each one.

Note: Any kind of sugar can be used if whizzed in the blender for a few seconds.

Eve's Fruit Cake

4 oz (115g) Barbados or soft brown sugar
4 oz (115g) vegan margarine softened at room temperature
½ lb (225g) plain wholemeal flour
1 level teaspoon cream of tartar
Rather less than 1 level teaspoon of bicarbonate of soda
1 heaped teaspoon cake spice (optional)
4 oz (115g) of any dried fruit
1 oz (30g) chopped peel
1 level teaspoon agar-agar
Water to mix

1. Cream together sugar and margarine. Sieve together flour, cream of tartar, bicarbonate of soda and cake spice and add to the creamed mixture, gradually.

2. Add fruit, dissolve agar-agar in a little water and mix in, adding water until just soft enough to beat. Beat for 2 or 3 minutes, put into a small cake tin and bake for 1 hour at 325°F/170°C (Gas Mark 3).

3. Cover with greaseproof paper and reduce heat to 250°F/130°C (Gas Mark ½) for a further 20-30 minutes. When cake stops 'singing' it is ready to be tested with a warm, dry knife or skewer which should leave the cake quite clean.

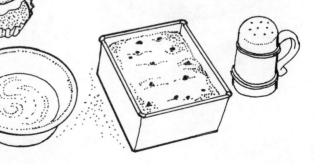

CHRISTMAS CAKE

2 lbs (900g) washed, dried fruit (raisins,
currants, sultanas)
1 pint (570ml) water
7 fl oz (200ml) vegetable oil
1 lb (455g) self-raising wholemeal flour
2 oz (55g) almonds, blanched and
chopped
1 tablespoon molasses
Rind of 1 lemon, grated
Pinch of spice

1. Mix all ingredients in order given.

2. Beat well and pour into well-lined,
greased 9-inch (23cm) cake tin and bake
for 2 hours at 300°F/150°C (Gas Mark 2).

3. Reduce heat to 250°F/130°C (Gas Mark
½) cover with greaseproof paper and
continue to cook for another 1½-2 hours.

CONNIE'S FRUIT CAKE

Skin and halve 1½ oz (45g) of almonds
Put into large saucepan —
½ pint (285ml) vegetable milk
concentrate (undiluted)
4 fl oz (115ml) water
½ lb (225g) margarine
6 oz (170g) Barbados sugar
1½ lbs (680g) mixed dried fruit (as
desired)

1. Mix all ingredients and bring to boil
stirring all the time, then simmer for 15
minutes.

2. Let it cool, then add grated rind of an
orange, pinch of salt, 1 level teaspoon
bicarbonate of soda and ¾ lb (340g)
wholemeal flour.

3. Mix well, turn into non-stick or well-
lined 8-inch (20cm) cake tin. Decorate top
with blanched almonds.

4. Bake in oven for 3 hours in all, 1 hour
at 325°F/170°C (Gas Mark 3), 2 hours at
275°F/140°C (Gas Mark 1). Cover top
with brown paper to prevent the nuts
burning.

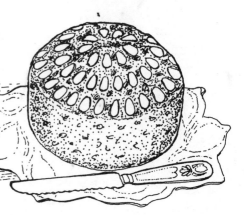

Fruit Cake with Carob

¾ lb (340g) wholemeal self-raising flour
6 fl oz (170ml) sunflower oil
(10 tablespoons)
1 tin carob milk concentrate
6 oz (170g) sultanas
2 tablespoons black treacle
Pinch of cinnamon

1. Mix all ingredients together and place in greased cake tin.

2. Bake for 1 hour at 350°F/180°C (Gas Mark 4).

Marzipan

6 oz (170g) ground almonds
2 oz (55g) soya flour
Juice and grated rind of 1 lemon
½ lb (225g) soft brown sugar
Almond essence

1. Mix nuts, flour and lemon rind. Add a few drops of almond essence and sufficient lemon juice to bind to a stiff consistency.

2. Cover the cake when cold and decorate.

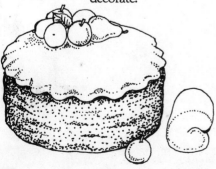

Festive Chocolate Sponge Cake

7 oz (200g) 81% self-raising flour
1 heaped teaspoon baking powder
1 oz (30g) cocoa or drinking chocolate
2 oz (55g) soft brown sugar
3 fl oz (90ml) oil
8 fl oz (230ml) water

Filling:
2 oz (55g) vegan margarine
2 oz (55g) finely ground Demerara sugar
2 oz (55g) apple, grated and mashed to a pulp
A little lemon juice

1. Mix dry ingredients.

2. Mix oil and water and stir into the dry ingredients and beat until smooth.

3. Cook in oiled sandwich tins for 15 minutes at 350°F/180°C (Gas Mark 4). Allow to cool before removing from tins.

4. Warm the margarine and beat to a cream with the sugar.

5. Beat in the apple with the lemon juice to prevent discoloration. Use to sandwich the sponge cakes together.

In place of eggs: To each ½ lb (225g) of flour add 1 teaspoon agar-agar dissolved in a little water to which a few drops of lemon juice have been added.

Note: As this cake contains raw fruit it should not be kept for more than a day or so.

Pastry, Biscuits and Cookies

1. The cooler the atmosphere, ingredients and utensils, as well as your hands, the lighter the pastry.
2. The less liquid and the more fat you use in shortcrust pastry, the shorter it will be.
3. Use a light touch when rolling out, and as little flour as possible. These pastry mixtures can be rolled out more easily if the pastry is placed between two sheets of greaseproof paper.
4. Take care not to stretch pastry when covering a pie plate, lining a flan ring or covering a pie dish. If you do, it will shrink from the edge.
5. Make a cross-cut in the centre of pies or tarts to allow the steam to escape.
6. Prick the bottom of lined pie plates or flan rings with a fork to allow air to escape while baking, or the case may be bumpy in centre.
7. Cooking: the average time to allow for shortcrust pastry is 30 minutes at 400°F/200°C (Gas Mark 6).
8. Wholemeal flour has a more crumbly texture than refined white from which the wheatgerm has been removed, and handles slightly differently. This is particularly noticeable when making pastry.
9. Cooks not accustomed to using 100% wholemeal flour in pastry making could try replacing a little of the wholemeal flour with 81% flour for a while.

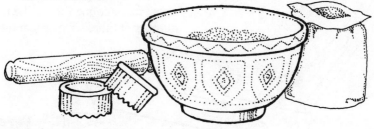

Quick Vegan Pastry

½ lb (225g) wholemeal flour
1 teaspoon baking powder
Pinch of salt (if to be used in savoury dish)
A little less than 5 dessertspoons vegetable oil
3-4 tablespoons cold water

1. Mix flour, baking powder and salt (if used).

2. Mix oil and water and add to the flour stirring lightly but thoroughly. Put in a cold place for at least 30 minutes.

3. Meanwhile prepare whatever filling is to be used.

4. Roll out pastry as required between two sheets of greaseproof paper. This will save a floury mess, sticky hands and help to stop pastry 'breaking' during handling.

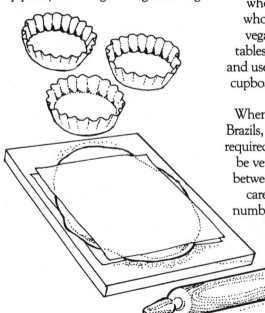

Wholemeal Pastry

½ lb (225g) wholemeal flour
Salt
2 oz (55g) vegan margarine
2 oz (55g) white fat
Cold water

1. Sieve the flour with a little salt. Rub in the fats until the mixture resembles breadcrumbs.

2. Add water, slowly mixing first with a knife. Knead lightly to a stiff dough. If not being used immediately, keep in a cool place, covered with a cloth.

Nut Pastry

To make nut pastry add 1½ oz (45g) of ground Brazil nuts to 4½ oz (130g) of wholemeal flour (or 100% and 81% wholemeal mixed). Rub in 2 oz (55g) vegan margarine. Mix with a bare 2 tablespoons of very cold water. Roll out and use as required. If returned to the cold cupboard for later use, cover with a cloth to prevent drying out.

When using nuts in pastry, particularly Brazils, less water and less fat than usual is required. Because the uncooked pastry will be very short, it is advisable to roll out between two sheets of kitchen foil, with careful handling this can be used a number of times for pastry and biscuits.

Short Pastry

Whenever possible use vegetable oil (natural polyunsaturated fat) rather than a hydrogenated (solid) fat for cooking. This quickest ever recipe for short pastry demonstrates how oil, as well as being nutritionally superior, has the added advantage of being more economical in use.

½ lb (225g) wholemeal flour
1 teaspoon baking powder
Pinch of salt
3 fl oz (90ml) oil
2-3 fl oz (60-90ml) water

1. Mix flour, baking powder and salt.

2. Stir in oil and water.

3. Mix lightly but thoroughly. Wrap and place in refrigerator or other very cool place until required. The mixture of wholemeal flour and oil make it necessary to use greaseproof paper or cooking foil when rolling out, but the resulting nutty flavour makes this little extra trouble well worth while. Particularly recommended for savoury tarts and pies. Excellent cold.

Quick Savoury Biscuits

½ lb mixed flours; equal quantities wheat flour, cornflour, rye flour, finely ground oats or muesli base (or any other mixture as desired)
8 tablespoons vegetable oil
4 tablespoons water
1 teaspoon yeast extract
A few cashew nuts

1. Heat oven to 300°F/150°C (Gas Mark 2).

2. Mix dry ingredients together.

3. Mix oil, water and yeast extract. Stir into dry ingredients and leave for a few minutes to thicken.

4. Take small pieces of the mixture, roll in the hands and flatten to biscuit size and shape. Place half a cashew nut on each. This should make about 30-34 2-inch (5cm) biscuits.

5. Bake low in the oven for 25-30 minutes. (If biscuits are not pressed quite so thin a longer baking time at a lower heat will be necessary.)

Note: This quick no-roll-out recipe can also be used for sweet biscuits. Simply replace the yeast extract with 1 tablespoon soft brown sugar and a pinch of allspice, cinnamon or ginger.

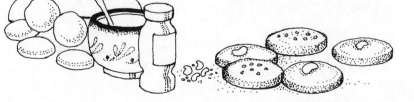

Classic Shortbread

6 oz (170g) wholemeal flour
4 oz (115g) vegan margarine
A few drops of vanilla flavouring
1 oz (30g) soft brown sugar
Pinch of salt

1. Knead all ingredients together into a ball.

2. When smooth, press into a greased, floured, 8-inch (20cm) baking tin. Pinch the edges and prick well with a fork.

3. Bake at 300°F/150°C (Gas Mark 2) for 20 minutes.

Note: Variations of this recipe include the addition of a few well-washed and dried raisins in place of the flavouring or 2 oz (55g) ground almonds or Brazil nuts.

Orange Oatcakes

4 oz (115g) vegan margarine
3 oz (85g) soft brown sugar
1 teaspoon syrup
1 tablespoon hot water
4 oz (115g) wholemeal flour
4 oz (115g) rolled oats
Grated rind of a good-sized orange

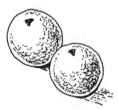

1. Cream together the fat, sugar and syrup.

2. Add the water, then stir in the flour and oats. When well mixed add the orange peel.

3. This can be cooked in a shallow tin and cut into squares when cold or made into small rocky cookies. For cookies put the mixture onto two greased oven trays in small heaps. Lightly flatten with a knife and leave reasonably thick. This quantity will make about 18 oatcakes. Cook at 350°F/180°C (Gas Mark 4) for 20-25 minutes.

Almond Toppers

1 oz (30g) whole almonds
5 oz (140g) vegan margarine
2 oz (55g) ground almonds
4 oz (115g) wholemeal flour
3 oz (85g) soft brown sugar

1. Scald and skin the whole almonds and split into halves.

2. Cream the margarine, stir in the ground almonds, then work in the flour and sugar gradually. Knead until smooth, roll out and cut into biscuits.

3. Put a piece of almond on each biscuit, leave to stand for a while in the cool to set the shapes well.

4. Bake at 350°F/180°C (Gas Mark 4) for 20-30 minutes according to thickness of biscuit. If this quantity is cut into 30 biscuits they will cook in 20 minutes.

GINGERNUTS

57.5 4 oz (115g) vegan margarine 38.3
42.5 3 oz (85g) golden syrup 28.3
3 oz (85g) soft brown sugar 26.3
112.5 ½ lb (225g) wholemeal flour 75
3 oz (85g) rolled oats 28.3
2 teaspoons ginger (ground) or a little less
Pinch of salt
1 teaspoon bicarbonate of soda

1. Put the margarine, syrup and sugar into a pan over very low heat.

2. In a separate bowl mix the flour, oats, ginger and salt.

3. Dissolve the bicarbonate of soda in a teaspoon of water and add to the warm mixture in the pan. Stir in the dry ingredients.

4. Drop small spoonfuls onto a greased baking tray leaving plenty of space between as the mixture will spread out to biscuit size.

5. Bake for 15-20 minutes at 325°F/170°C (Gas Mark 3).

CALIFORNIA ORANGE COOKIES

3 oz (85g) Barbados sugar
5 oz (140g) vegan margarine
3 oz (85g) wholemeal flour
1½ oz (45g) wheatgerm flakes
2 teaspoons lemon juice
1½ oz (45g) soya flour
1 tablespoon grated orange rind
4 oz (115g) ground almonds

1. Cream sugar and margarine.

2. Add the rest of the ingredients and mix well.

3. Mould into smooth shape and leave wrapped in foil for an hour to firm. Roll out carefully between sheets of film into not-too-thin biscuits.

4. Cut into shape and bake on a greased baking tray at 350°F/180°C (Gas Mark 4) for 20 minutes.

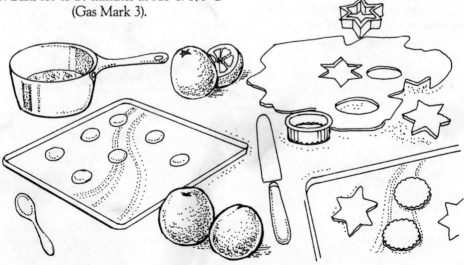

Cinnamon Biscuits

3 oz (85g) vegan margarine
2 oz (55g) Barbados sugar (or 1½ oz/45g fruit sugar)
6 oz (170g) wholemeal flour (or 5 oz/140g flour and 1 oz/30g soya wheatgerm and soya flour mixed)
1 heaped teaspoon ground cinnamon
A little cold water

1. Heat oven to 350°F/180°C (Gas Mark 4). Lightly oil and flour baking trays (if not non-stick).

2. Thoroughly cream together margarine and sugar.

3. Sieve together dry ingredients and work these into the cream a little at a time, adding a spoonful or two of water if necessary. When it will all hold together, knead for 2 or 3 minutes.

4. Roll out very thinly between two sheets of transparent cooking foil (lightly sprinkle with flour if inclined to stick).

5. Cut into 2 inch (5cm) biscuits, prick, and bake in a lower half of oven for 10 to 12 minutes. If biscuits are soft in centre after this time they can go back for a couple of minutes to dry out, and the next batch must be rolled out more thinly.

Note: Biscuit making is not really difficult. After a very little experimenting with rolling out and finding the shelves in your own oven which give the best results, you will be able to produce a batch of 60-80 delicous biscuits quickly and be certain of excellent results every time. For variety cinnamon can be replaced by ginger, coconut, vanilla or other flavours.

Oatmeal Shortbread

4 oz (115g) wholemeal flour
2 oz (55g) medium oatmeal
4 oz (115g) vegan margarine
2 oz (55g) Barbados sugar

1. Put all ingredients into mixing bowl and knead together into adhesive ball.

2. Press into sandwich tin, level with a fork and prick. Bake at 400°F/200°C (Gas Mark 6) for 20-25 minutes.

Carob Shortcake Biscuits

3 oz (85g) wholemeal flour
2 oz (55g) vegan margarine
1 oz (30g) carob flour
1 oz (30g) soya flour
1 oz (30g) soft brown sugar

1. Mix all ingredients and knead to a smooth texture.

2. Roll out between 2 sheets of clear cooking foil.

3. Cut into shapes, prick with a fork and bake for 10 minutes at 325°F/170°C (Gas Mark 3) on a greased baking sheet.

Barley Nibbles

1½ oz (45g) vegan margarine
1 tablespoon syrup
1 tablespoon soft brown sugar
4 oz (115g) barley kernels
Vanilla essence or grated rind of 1 lemon

1. Warm the fat and syrup in a pan, stir in the sugar until dissolved. Remove from the heat and stir in the barley kernels and flavouring.

2. Mix thoroughly, pressing the ingredients together.

3. Drop small spoonfuls onto a well greased baking tin and cook for 25-30 minutes at 350°F/180°C (Gas Mark 4).

Hazelnut Shortbread

3 oz (85g) vegan margarine
3 oz (85g) wholemeal self-raising flour
2 oz (55g) soft light brown sugar
2 oz (55g) milled hazelnuts

1. Rub fat into flour to make a crumble. Work in sugar and hazelnuts and knead the mixture lightly.

2. Prepare a well-greased greaseproof sheet to cover shallow baking tin.

3. Press mixture into tin and bake in slow oven, middle shelf, 300°F/150°C (Gas Mark 2) for 30 minutes, but after 15 minutes remove from oven and mark into portions and replace in oven for remaining fifteen minutes.

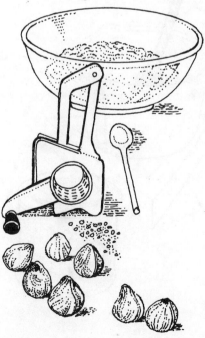

EVA'S PARKIN

6 oz (170g) treacle
3 oz (85g) vegan margarine
½ lb (225g) wholemeal flour
3 oz (85g) Barbados sugar
½ oz (15g) cake spice, ginger and nutmeg,
mixed
4 oz (115g) rolled oats

1. Warm treacle in heavy-based saucepan.

2. Rub fat into flour, add sugar, spice and oats. Add this to the warmed treacle and mix thoroughly.

3. Press into greased, flat shallow tin.

4. Bake for 15 minutes at 350°F/180°C (Gas Mark 4). When cooked, cut into strips and leave to cool.

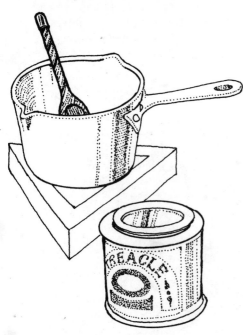

PAT'S FLAPJACKS

5 oz (140g) vegan margarine
6 oz (170g) Barbados sugar
9 oz (255g) rolled oats
Pinch of salt

1. Warm margarine in large saucepan and when melted stir in sugar. Mix well, then stir in oats and salt.

2. Grease a swiss roll tin and press mixture into this making the surface level.

3. Bake at 325°F/170°C (Gas Mark 3) for 30 minutes in centre of oven. Remove from heat and mark into biscuit-sized pieces, but leave in the tin until cool.

COCONUT CRISP

4 oz (115g) cashew or nut cream
2 oz (55g) crushed wheatflakes
1 oz (30g) Barbados sugar
4 oz (115g) wholemeal flour
3 oz (85g) desiccated coconut

1. Warm margarine gently and mix in the other ingredients.

2. Knead well and press into well-greased baking tin and bake for 10 minutes at 325°F/170°C (Gas Mark 3).

3. Mark into biscuits and return to the oven for a further 5-10 minutes. Leave in the tin to cool.

Flapjacks

4 oz (115g) brown sugar
4 oz (115g) vegan margarine
3 oz (85g) syrup
½ lb (225g) rolled oats

1. Mix and heat the sugar, margarine, and syrup.

2. Add oats and press into greased baking tin large enough to make the flapjacks quite thin.

3. Bake in pre-heated oven for 20-25 minutes at 350°F/180°C (Gas Mark 4). Cool for 5 mins before cutting into squares, but leave in tin until quite cool.

Oat Macaroons

3 oz (85g) vegan margarine
1½ oz (45g) brown sugar
1 (bare) tablespoon syrup
Almond essence
3 oz (85g) rolled oats
3 oz (85g) wholemeal flour
½ teaspoon baking powder
Pinch of salt

1. Cream the fat and sugar together until light, then work in the syrup and flavouring.

2. Separately mix the dry ingredients and gradually work this into the sugar mixture.

3. Divide into about 30 pieces and flatten into 2 inch rounds on a greased baking sheet.

4. Bake at 375°F/190°C (Gas Mark 5) for 10-12 minutes.

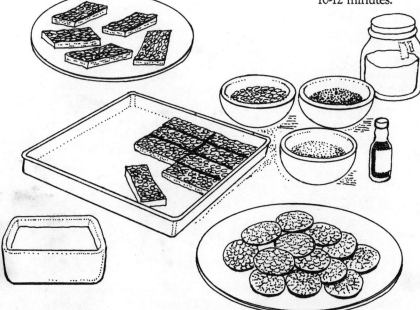

MISCELLANEOUS

APRICOT MINCEMEAT

1 lb (455g) good quality apricots
1 lb (455g) apples
1 lb (455g) dates
1 lb (455g) raisins
1 lb (455g) currants
1 lb (455g) vegetable suet
1 lb (455g) sugar
2 oz (60g) chopped almonds
½ oz (15g) grated nutmeg
Grated rind and juice of 1 large lemon

1. Soak the apricots overnight in very little water, drain, then chop.

2. Chop the apples, the dates and raisins. Mix together adding the currants, suet, sugar, almonds, nutmeg and lemon.

3. Mix well, pack into clean, dry jars, leaving a space at the top. Seal with a cellophane disc, then cover with paper circles and tie down.

Note: Do not use waxed paper seals, as the wax may not be vegan.

RAW MARMALADE
(Yields 4½ Jars)

½ lb (225g) apricots
3 or 4 oranges
2 lemons
2 lb (490g) sugar

1. Soak the apricots overnight. Drain, and mince with the peeled oranges. Use only 3 oranges if they are juicy, to prevent the marmalade ending up too runny. Mince the lemons, and stir in the sugar. Leave 30 minutes.

2. Mix in a blender for 5 minutes until the sugar has dissolved. Do not overblend.

3. Pack into clean, dry jars, seal with cellophane discs, and cover.

Plamil and Banana Shake

1 banana
1 teaspoon sugar
½ pint (285ml) vegetable milk
A little cinnamon (optional)

1. Liquidize banana and sugar. Whisk in *Plamil* and serve. Almost any fresh fruit can be used in place of the banana; a very pleasant shake is made with dried, soaked apricots.

Treacle Toffee Apples

1 lb (455g) Barbados sugar
4 level tablespoons West Indian black treacle
4 tablespoons water
8 medium apples

1. Bring sugar, black treacle and water to boil slowly to dissolve the sugar.

2. Then boil rapidly for 5 minutes — or to 310°F/155°C — when the syrup will form a firm ball if dropped into cold water.

3. Stick apples securely on wooden skewers and coat with the toffee. Place on oiled greaseproof paper and allow to set.

Altogether Cake

6 oz (170g) mixed dried fruit (apricots, prunes, sultanas, raisins)
2 oz (55g) stoned dates
4 oz (115g) coconut
4 oz (115g) rice flour
4 oz (115g) ground sunflower seeds (or nuts)
1 teaspoon mixed spice
1 large apple
1 tablespoon sunflower seed oil
7 tablespoons water

1. Wash fruit including dates and soak in hot water for 20 minutes.

2. Meanwhile, mix coconut, rice flour, seeds and spice.

3. Chop the soaked fruit (when soft but not soggy) with apples and mix into dry ingredients. Stir in oil and water and mix well.

4. Press into baking tray and leave to set in cold place. Cut into small squares. A great favourite.

Apple and Barley Water

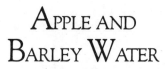

2 apples (medium)
1½ pints (850ml) water
2 tablespoons barley kernels
Flavouring such as cloves, ginger or cinnamon

1. Wash and chop the apples with core and peel.

2. Place all in a saucepan with the barley kernels and simmer with the flavouring for half an hour.

3. Strain, sweeten to taste and set aside to cool.

LEMONADE

2 tablespoons barley kernels
2 tablespoons Barbados sugar
Juice of ½ lemon and the pared rind
1 pint (570ml) boiling water

1. Place the barley kernels in a jug, add the sugar, lemon juice and rind.

2. Pour the boiling water over it and allow to stand until cold. Strain.

FRUIT BARLEY WATER

½ lb (225g) blackcurrants or raspberries
3 pints (1.7l) water
2 oz (55g) barley kernels
Sugar to taste

1. Stew the fruit in water until the juice is extracted, strain and squeeze the fruit to remove as much juice as possible.

2. Add the barley kernels and sugar and re-boil gently, stirring occasionally. Serve hot or cold.

PINEAPPLE COLESLAW

Pineapple juice
French Dressing
Shredded white cabbage
Red unpeeled apple, chopped
Pineapple chunks
A little chopped celery
Lettuce leaves

1. Mix the pineapple juice with the French dressing, blending well.

2. Toss with the cabbage, apple, pineapple and celery.

3. Serve in a bowl lined with lettuce leaves. Quantities to taste.

VEGETABLE CREAM CHEESE

To ¾ pint (425ml) of concentrated vegetable milk (sugar-free or original) add a quarter pint of water. Heat and watch carefully. As it begins to rise in pan, remove from heat and stir in the juice of two medium-sized lemons (one and a half if they are extra juicy). It will begin to curdle immediately. Pour into cheese cloth and hang to drip overnight or for several hours. Turn into dish, add dessertspoon vegetable oil, sea salt and flavouring. This can be fresh chives finely chopped, celery seed, or any herb your family enjoys. Serve on dry biscuits, in salads or use to top 'Crisp and Nutties.'

This cheese can also be made with soya flour, using 2 oz (55g) dry vegetable milk to a little less than ½ pint of water. Proceed as above.

Soya 'Cheese' (Cream Style)

4 oz (115g) soya flour
Yeast extract to taste
2 fl oz (60ml) vegetable oil

Mix well and leave to set. Store in cool place. Fresh herbs could be used for flavouring in place of the yeast extract but if so the cheese should be used within a day or two.

Soya 'Cheese' (Cheddar Style)

3½ oz (100g) *Soyolk* or other heat-treated soya flour
1 good teaspoon yeast extract or to taste
4 oz (115g) vegan margarine

Melt margarine, stir in flour and yeast extract. Beat until smooth and leave to set.

'Cheese' Snacks. Put slices of soya cheese on toasted bread and grill until the cheese melts and crispens. Serve with sliced tomatoes and parsley for a well-balanced meal.

'Cheese' Sweethearts. Put slices of 'cheese' between slices of wholemeal bread and shallow fry in vegetable oil until both sides are crisp and the 'cheese' has melted. Serve as above.

Soya Compote

1 oz (30g) raisins
2 fl oz (60ml) vegetable oil
¼ pint (140ml) vegetable milk, or a little more
2 oz (55g) soya flakes
1 oz (30g) dried apricots
2 oz (55g) finely chopped nuts

1. Soak the raisins for 1 hour or more.

2. Chop the apricots, mix the soya flakes into the oil, add the raisins, nuts and milk.

3. Bake in an oiled dish for 40 minutes at 350°F/180°C (Gas Mark 5).

4. Serve hot or cold with a vegan cream.

Carob Drink

Take 1 pint soya milk, sweeten and flavour to taste with carob powder. Heated it makes a warming drink. For a refreshing cold drink try the addition of orange juice in place of the carob.

CONTRIBUTIONS FROM DORIS AND VI

MUSHROOM SOUP

1 tablespoon vegetable oil
2 medium onions
4 oz (115g) mushrooms
1 pint (570ml) vegetable stock
2 tablespoons soya flour
2 teaspoons cornflour

1. Heat oil in pan and gently fry chopped onions and mushrooms.

2. Add stock and simmer for about 30 minutes.

3. Mix soya flour and cornflour with a little cold water and add to soup then bring to the boil for a further 10 minutes.

VEGETABLE SOUP

1 pint (570ml) vegetable stock
2 sticks celery
2 medium carrots
2 medium onions
1 parsnip
1 turnip
Yeast extract for flavouring

1. Put vegetable stock in pan and bring to the boil.

2. Chop or mince all vegetables, add to the stock and simmer for about 30 minutes.

3. Add yeast extract about 10 minutes before serving.

ONION SOUP

1 pint (570ml) vegetable stock
1 lb (455g) onions
2 medium potatoes
2 tablespoons soya flour
1 tablespoon cornflour

1. Put vegetable stock in pan and bring to the boil.

2. Chop or mince onions and potatoes. Add to the stock and simmer for about 30 minutes.

3. Mix soya flour and cornflour with a little cold water and add about 10 minutes before serving.

APPLE ROLYPOLY

3 oz (85g) vegan margarine
6 oz (170g) wholemeal self-raising flour
1 tablespoon red jam
2 medium apples
Raw cane sugar

1. Rub fat into flour, mix with a little cold water and roll into an oblong shape.

2. Spread with jam and sliced apples, sprinkle with sugar and roll, sealing ends.

3. Place in oven dish and bake at 400°F/200°C (Gas Mark 6) until pale brown. Sprinkle with sugar.

Eggless Fruit Cake

¾ lb (340g) wholemeal flour
A good pinch of salt
¼ level teaspoon ground cinnamon
¼ level teaspoon ground nutmeg
½ level teaspoon mixed spice
1½ oz (45g) vegan margarine
½ lb (225g) soft brown sugar
½ lb (225g) cleaned sultanas
5 oz (140g) stoneless raisins
6 oz (170g) washed currants
1 oz (30g) finely chopped candied peel
2 oz (55g) glacé cherries, quartered
Finely grated rind of 1 lemon
½ pint (295ml) water
¾ level teaspoon barcarbonate of soda

1. Grease a cake tin and line it with greaseproof paper to come an inch (2.5cm) above the sides of the tin. Brush the paper with melted fat.

2. Sift together the flour, salt, cinnamon, nutmeg and mixed spice. Rub in the margarine, then mix in the brown sugar.

3. Mix all the fruit with the grated lemon rind and stir it into the mixture.

4. Make a hollow in the centre, pour in all but two tablespoonsful of the water and stir in lightly.

5. Warm the two tablespoons water slightly and pour it over the bicarbonate of soda, then stir it thoroughly into the mixture, without actually beating.

6. Turn the mixture into the prepared tin. Bake the cake in a moderate oven, about 350°F/180°C (Gas Mark 4) for an hour then reduce the heat to 325°F/170°C (Gas Mark 3) for a further hour or until the cake is cooked.

Tea Cake

2 oz (55g) stoned dates
4 oz (115g) mixed fruit
1 oz (30g) mixed peel
¼ pint (140ml) strained cold tea
2 oz (55g) Demerara sugar
2 oz (55g) vegan margarine
1 tablespoon golden syrup
8 oz (225g) wholemeal self-raising flour
1 level teaspoon bicarbonate of soda
2 fl oz (60ml) soya milk

1. Grease and line a 7-inch (18cm) round deep cake tin with greased greaseproof paper.

2. Chop the dates and place in pan with mixed dried fruits, peel, tea, sugar, margarine and syrup. Bring to simmering point and allow to simmer for 3 minutes. Remove from heat and allow mixture to cool.

3. When cold gradually mix in the sifted flour and bicarbonate of soda which has been dissolved in warm soya milk.

4. Mix thoroughly and turn into a prepared tin.

5. Bake in the centre of a moderately slow oven 325°F/170°C (Gas Mark 3) for 1¼ hours. Allow the cake to cook a little before removing from tin.

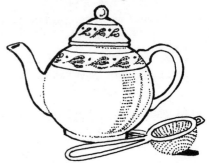

ALMOND CRUNCHY CAKES

½ oz (15g) whole almonds
6 oz (170g) vegan margarine
4 oz (115g) Demarara sugar
2 tablespoons golden syrup
½ lb (225g) quick oats
Large pinch of salt
1 oz (30g) flaked almonds

1. Heat oven to 375°F/190°C (Gas Mark 5). Grease two round 7-inch (18cm) sponge tins. Line the bases with greaseproof paper.

2. Put the whole almonds in a pan with just enough water to cover and bring to boil. Run the nuts under a cold tap, remove the skins. Slice each nut in half.

3. Melt margarine in a pan with the sugar and syrup. Stir in oats, salt and flaked almonds. Mix together.

4. Divide the mixture between the two tins. Smooth the tops. Arrange nuts round the top.

5. Bake in centre of preheated oven for 20 minutes or until golden. Cool in the tins. Cut each round into six.

RASPBERRY BUNS

½ lb (225g) wholemeal self-raising flour
Pinch of salt
3 oz (85g) vegan margarine
3 oz (85g) brown sugar
3-4 tablespoons soya milk
jam

1. Heat oven to 375°F/190°C (Gas Mark 5). Grease baking tray.

2. Sift flour and salt, rub in fat, add sugar.

3. Mix together thoroughly, add milk to make stiff dough.

4. Turn on to floured board and form roll. Cut off pieces ¾-inch (2cm) thick and place on baking tray.

5. Make a hollow in centre of each, fill with jam. Brush round edges with soya milk and bake for 15-20 minutes until golden brown.

JAM OR SYRUP SPONGE PUDDING

2 tablespoons jam
3 oz (85g) vegan margarine
6 oz (170g) wholemeal self-raising flour

1. Grease pudding basin and put syrup or jam in the bottom.

2. Rub fat into flour and mix to a stiff consistency with water.

3. Place mixture in basin on top of jam, cover with foil and steam 1½-2 hours.

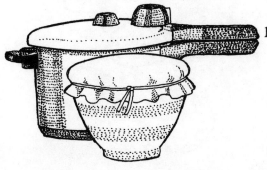

Mabel's Recipes

All flour is 100 per cent wholemeal unless otherwise stated.

All sugar is Barbados.

Oil is either sunflower or soya but any other would do.

Wholemeal Bread

1½ lb (680g) stoneground wholemeal flour
4 oz (115g) soya flour
1 heaped teaspoon sea salt
1 oz (30g) fresh yeast (or ½ oz/15g dried)
About 1 pint (570ml) lukewarm water

1. Mix dry ingredients. Whisk yeast in a little of the water and pour into well in the flour. Add remaining water and mix thoroughly; first with a spoon and then kneading slightly by hand.

2. Form into two small loaves, using a little more flour if the mixture has been too wet. Experience will tell just how much water is needed; the exact quantity varies with different flours.

3. Place in greased tins and leave in a warm place to rise for about 15 minutes, covering with a cloth or putting in a polythene bag. Bake 1 hour. Temperature about 400°F/200°C (Gas Mark 6) to commence; then allow to fall to 350°F/180°C (Gas Mark 4).

Fruit Loaf

Make dough to above recipe but using only half quantity. Add 3 oz (85g) raw cane sugar, 2 oz (85g) white fat and 4 oz (115g) of any dried fruits, also a little spice if liked. Allow a little longer time for rising than for the bread; if you have plenty of time it can be left to rise 15 minutes before shaping; then knead slightly, put in tin and leave a further 10 minutes.

Bake at 425°F/220°C (Gas Mark 7) for 10 minutes, then reduce heat to 350°F/180°C (Gas Mark 4) for another 35-40 minutes.

Plain Teacakes

To half above quantity of bread dough add two tablespoons oil and knead well into the dough. Form into small cakes and leave in a warm place (covered) until they are nearly double the size. Bake on greased baking sheet half an hour at 425°F/220°C (Gas Mark 7).

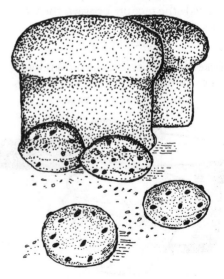

Pizza Dough

14 oz (395g) wholemeal flour
1 rounded teaspoon sea salt
1½ oz (45g) soya flour
½ oz (15g) fresh yeast
About ½ pint (285ml) lukewarm water
1 tablespoon oil

1. Mix dry ingredients.

2. Blend yeast in half a teacupful of the water and add to the flour with sufficient additional water to bind. Add oil and knead to a soft dough.

3. Cover and leave in a warm place for two or three hours; knead lightly before using.

Coblets

1. Take pizza dough and form into long, thin rolls about 1 inch (2.5cm) in diameter.

2. Cut diagonally across, forming triangles. These should be as small as possible.

3. Bake twelve minutes in a very hot oven 450°F/230°C (Gas Mark 8). Serve with soup or as a buffet snack.

Plain Scones
(This quantity makes 20)

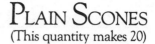

1¼ lb (565g) wholemeal flour
2 oz (55g) soya flour
½ teaspoon sea salt (could be a little more if desired)
1½ level teaspoons cream of tartar
Just over 1 level teaspoon bicarbonate of soda
5 oz (140g) vegan margarine
Cold water for binding

1. Mix all ingredients and rub into fat. Bind with cold water.

2. Roll out not more than 1 inch (2.5cm) thick and cut into rounds.

3. Bake at about 450°F/230°C (Gas Mark 8) for about 20 minutes.

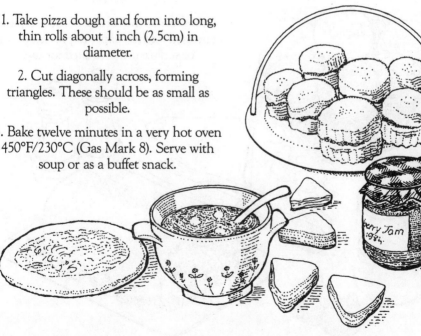

Wholemeal Rolls

¾ lb (340g) wholemeal flour
2 oz (55g) soya flour
1 level teaspoon sea salt
½ oz (15g) fresh yeast
About ½ pint (285ml) warm water
1 tablespoon oil

1. Mix flours and salt thoroughly. Whisk yeast in a little of the water and pour into a well in the flour. Gradually add remaining water and finally oil.

2. Knead slightly and leave in a warm place in polythene bag for 20-30 minutes.

3. Re-knead on floured board; divide into eight rolls and leave to rise 15 minutes. Bake 35 minutes at 425°F/220°C (Gas Mark 7).

Savoury Onion Sauce

1 medium onion
2 tablespoons oil
1 level teaspoon basil, sage or marjoram
½ pint (285ml) vegetable stock
2 level tablespoons fine oatmeal
2 level tablespoons soya flour
A good heaped teaspoon yeast extract

1. Dice onion and cook in oil until soft. Add herbs and stir. Add stock.

2. Mix oatmeal and soya flour and stir smoothly with a little cold water. Pour into this some of the boiling liquid and stir. Return to the pan while stirring vigorously, add yeast extract and stir gently until the sauce reaches boiling point.

3. Press on to the surface of sauce a piece of greased kitchen paper to prevent drying of surface until required for use.

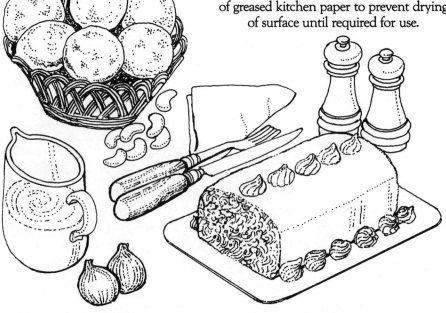

Butter Bean Surprise

1 oz (30g) tvp
1 teaspoon yeast extract
1 clove garlic, crushed
1 pint (570ml) water
6 oz brown rice
3 tablespoons oil
2 cloves
1 bay leaf
Freshly ground black pepper
1 teaspoon sea salt
3 oz (85g) soya flour
1 tablespoon tomato purée
11 oz (310g) can whole-style sweetcorn
3 oz (85g) coarsely chopped olives
white fat

1. Place tvp in basin with yeast extract, crushed garlic and 8 fl oz (230ml) hot water.

2. Stir rice in oil over heat 5 minutes. Add tvp, 1 pint (570ml) water and seasoning, and cook for a further 20 minutes.

3. Stir in soya flour, tomato purée, corn and olives.

4. Shape, cover with bean paste (recipe below) dot with fat and bake for 40 minutes at 350°F/180°C (Gas Mark 4).

Bean coating for above:
½ lb (225g) soaked skinned butter beans
½ pint (285ml) cold water
½ teaspoon sea salt
Freshly ground black pepper
1 level teaspoon powdered caraway
1 level teaspoon powdered cumin
1 oz (30g) white fat

1. Cook beans in water, add salt, pepper, spices and fat.
2. Stir over low heat until fairly stiff. Sieve.

Festive Roast

1 medium sized onion
2 fl oz (60ml) vegetable oil
1 tablespoon dried marjoram (or basil, sage or savoury)
A pinch of salt
1 good teaspoon yeast extract
Water to mix
6 oz (170g) wholemeal bread
3 oz (85g) milled Brazils
3 oz (85g) milled hazels
1 oz (30g) wholemeal flour
1 oz (30g) soya flour
1 large chopped pepper
2 oz (55g) milled cashews
2 tablespoons oil
Macaroni
Celery leaves or parsley

1. Chop onion finely and cook in oil until nearly brown. Add herbs, sea salt, yeast extract and about a teacupful boiling water. Stir, then pour on to bread which has been broken down into small pieces.

2. Weigh Brazil and hazelnuts, flour and soya flour and mix together.

3. By this time the bread should be soaked enough to mash down. Add nuts and flours and stir vigorously until mixture is smooth and free from lumps. If too dry, a little more water may be needed but mixture should be quite stiff.

4. Spread half mixture on baking sheet, cover with chopped pepper and then a further layer of nutmeat. Shape.

5. Mix two ounces milled cashews with two tablespoons oil and force through piping bag to make decorative rosettes on the roast. Bake for ¾ hour at 400°F/200°C (Gas Mark 6).

6. Cook wholemeal macaroni in boiling water for twenty minutes. When roast is cooked decorate with pieces of macaroni.

7. Coat the roast with the following glaze, using a teaspoon. Garnish with celery leaves or parsley.

GLAZE FOR ROAST

8 fl oz (230ml) hot water
½ level teaspoon powdered agar agar
1 small teaspoon yeast extract

1. Bring water almost to the boil, then commence sprinkling on agar powder very gradually while still on heat, stirring thoroughly and vigorously.

2. When agar is thoroughly dissolved remove from heat and stir in yeast extract. While still hot, pour a spoonful at a time over nut roast until completely covered.

LENTIL AND TOMATO SAVOURY

6 oz (170g) red lentils
¾ pint (425ml) water
1 bay leaf
½ teaspoon marjoram
1 medium sized onion, diced
1 heaped teaspoon yeast extract
½ lb (225g) tomatoes, sliced
2 oz (55g) wholemeal breadcrumbs
1 tablespoon oil

1. Pick over and wash lentils and cook gently in the water with bay leaf, marjoram, diced onion and yeast extract for about 20 minutes until soft.

2. Grease a pie dish and make alternate layers of sliced tomato and lentil mixture, finishing with the latter and topping with oiled crumbs.

3. Bake half an hour until brown at 375°F/190°C (Gas Mark 5).

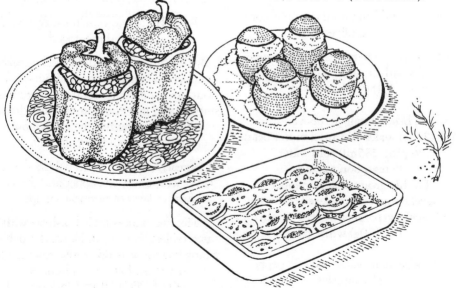

Stuffed Peppers

2 medium sized peppers
1 small tin whole sweetcorn
1 teaspoon wholemeal flour
A little thyme
2 teaspoons vegetable oil
Tinned soya beans
Also cooked brown rice and sliced shallots dipped in oil for a few hours, to garnish.

1. Wash peppers and carefully cut out stalk so that it can be replaced neatly. Remove seeds.

2. Drain sweetcorn and mix liquid with flour. Add thyme and oil, then the corn and an equal quantity (by volume) of tinned soya beans, or alternatively, Lima or haricot beans previously cooked in salted water.

3. Slowly heat these ingredients in a saucepan to almost boiling point, stirring to prevent sticking.

4. Fill peppers with mixture, replace stalk, place in greased dish, pour a few drops of oil over each and bake at once for about 35 minutes at 375°F/190°C (Gas Mark 5).

5. Place on a bed of rice garnished with the rings of shallot and sprigs of herb and serve with savoury rice.

Stuffed Tomatoes

Tomatoes
1 tablespoon ground cashews
1 tablespoon dried wholemeal breadcrumbs
2 good pinches curry powder

1. Scald and skin tomatoes if desired. Halve each tomato and remove pulp.

2. Mix nuts, wholemeal breadcrumbs and curry powder and stuff tomato cases, with this mixture.

3. Garnish and serve on lettuce leaves sprinkled with chopped chives, or on watercress.

Nut Rissoles

4 oz (115g) wholemeal breadcrumbs
4 oz (115g) grated onion
1 teaspoon basil
2 oz (55g) ground cashews
2 oz (55g) ground hazelnuts
1 oz (30g) wholemeal flour
1 oz (30g) soya flour
1 teaspoon yeast extract
A little sea salt
Hot water to mix

1. Crumble wholemeal bread and add grated onion and basil. Mix nuts, flour and soya flour.

2. Dissolve yeast extract and salt in a little hot water, then combine all ingredients. Mix thoroughly.

3. Form into rissoles, coat with flour and fry in oil until brown.

Mincemeat

½ lb (225g) currants
½ lb (225g) sultanas
½ lb (225g) raisins
4 oz (115g) mixed chopped peel
1 heaped teaspoon mixed spice
Juice and rind of 1 lemon
1 lb (455g) Barbados sugar
6 oz (170g) vegetable fat or oil
½ lb (225g) Bramley apples

1. Wash and dry fruit. Mix spice and lemon rind in sugar. Add dried fruits, lemon juice and fat.

2. Grate in apple, cored but not peeled. Stir well.

3. Allow to stand at least one day before potting, meanwhile keeping covered and stirring now and again. During this time the dried fruit will absorb surplus juice.

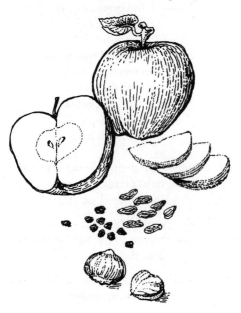

Durlston Pudding

1 oz (30g) chopped or broken cashews
1 tablespoon oil
2 heaped tablespoons marmalade
1 oz (30g) seedless raisins or sultanas
2 teaspoons hot water
3 oz (85g) unsweetened wheat flakes or other crisp cereal flakes

1. Brown nuts in oil; do not burn. Add marmalade, raisins, and hot water. Stir over heat for about 1 minute.

2. Allow to cool a little, then mix in wheat flakes.

3. Put in greased pie dish for 20 minutes, oven 325°F/170°C (Gas Mark 3). Serve with a soya custard or nut cream.

Lemon Nut Shortbread

3 oz (85g) flour
3 oz (85g) maizemeal
3 oz (85g) ground hazels
1 heaped tablespoon syrup
3 tablespoons lemon juice
3 oz (85g) vegan margarine

Mix all ingredients together, press out into shallow tins. Bake 30 minutes at 350°F/180°C (Gas Mark 4).

Chocolate Moulds

15 fl oz (230ml) soya milk
2 level teaspoons powdered agar-agar
1 rounded tablespoon cocoa
1 heaped tablespoon Barbados sugar

1. Bring milk to the boil, sprinkle on agar-agar very gradually, stirring briskly all the while until dissolved.

2. In a separate basin mix cocoa and sugar. Add to the agar solution and stir again while it slowly comes to the boil. Pour out and allow to cool.

3. Top with a good spoonful of jam, rosehip syrup, maple syrup or ground nuts.

Jellies

Agar-agar is the easiest thing to use for vegetarian jellies. The powdered form is most convenient. Use one level teaspoonful to each ½ pint (285ml) of liquid. Bring liquid to simmering point and sprinkle agar powder on very gradually, whisking meanwhile to prevent lumps forming. In a few minutes it will be dissolved. Add any flavouring desired and pour out to cool.

Fruit jellies: Take 1 pint of any fruit stock and sweeten to taste. Mix in 1½ heaped teaspoons of agar-agar and bring almost to the boil, then add ½ pint (285ml) of richly flavoured natural fruit juice, stir well together and pour into dish to set; or pour over stale cake to make a popular trifle, and top with milled nuts.

Coconut Milk

This is an excellent milk and well worth the trouble to make. Pour out and retain the liquid from the nut. Grate the white flesh of the coconut in a blender. Cover with boiling water and leave for 30 minutes or more. Strain through muslin and press out all the liquid. Add the water from the nut and use as a drink, or in place of milk for cooking.

Fruit Turnover

3 oz (85g) currants
3 oz (85g) sultanas
1 oz (30g) chopped peel
1 oz (30g) milled cashews
1 oz (30g) chopped cashews
1 oz (30g) Barbados sugar
1 tablespoon lemon juice

1. Mix all the ingredients together with large fork or pastry blender.

2. Roll out a square of wholemeal pastry and cover a little less than one half with the mixture.

3. Moisten edges, fold over and seal. Bake ½ hour at 450°F/230°C (Gas Mark 8).

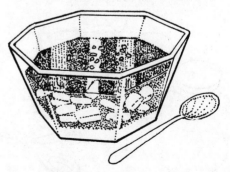

CAKES

Wholemeal flour can be used in most cake recipes and is, in fact, a great improvement in many cases as regards texture. Those who value their health will always choose stoneground, 100 per cent wholemeal flour.

COOKSON CAKE

½ lb (225g) wholemeal flour
4 oz (115g) raw sugar
½ teaspoon bicarbonate of soda
¾ teaspoon cream of tartar
½ teaspoon ground nutmeg
A good pinch of sea salt
4 oz (115g) white fat
2 oz (55g) seedless raisins
2 oz (55g) chopped peel
1 heaped tablespoon syrup

1. Mix dry ingredients and rub in fat. Then add raisins, chopped peel and syrup.

2. Add sufficient water to make mixture easy to beat. Beat well.

3. Put in greased shallow tin lined with greaseproof paper and bake for 40 minutes at 400°F/200°C (Gas Mark 6).

PARKIN

6 oz (170g) white fat
6 oz (170g) medium oatmeal
2 oz (55g) fine oatmeal
3 oz (85g) wholemeal flour
1 oz (30g) 81% flour
3 oz (85g) raw cane sugar
2 oz (55g) soya flour
2 teaspoons ground ginger
½ level teaspoon mixed spice
½ teaspoon sea salt
1 level teaspoon cream of tartar
Scant level teaspoon bicarbonate of soda
5 oz (140g) black treacle

1. Rub fat into dry ingredients. Add treacle and sufficient water to beat. Beat well.

2. Grease and line a flat baking tin with greaseproof paper. Bake for about 1¼ hours, 400°F/200°C (Gas Mark 6) to commence, allow to drop to 350°F/180°C (Gas Mark 4). Keep in tin for one week before cutting.

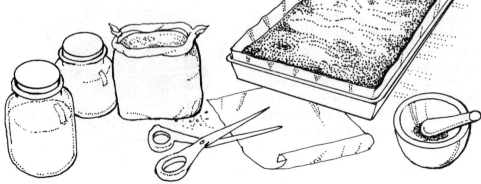

TWELFTH NIGHT CAKE

4 oz (115g) Barbados sugar
3 oz (85g) vegetarian fat
4½ oz (130g) wholemeal flour
1 oz (30g) soya flour
1 oz (30g) fine oatmeal
½ level teaspoon mixed spice
3 level tablespoons ground cashews
creamed with a small teacupful cold
water
1 tablespoon lemon juice
1 level teaspoon cream of tartar
¾ level teaspoon bicarbonate of soda

1. Beat together sugar and fat.

2. Mix wholemeal flour, soya flour,
oatmeal and mixed spice together in a
bowl.

3. Add to the mixture a little at a time,
alternating with the creamed cashew
mixture. Beat well.

4. Beat in the lemon juice, then fold in the
cream of tartar and bicarbonate of soda.

5. Divide between two sandwich tins and
bake for ¾ hour at 400°F/200°C (Gas
Mark 6). When cold sandwich the cake
with home-made mincemeat and decorate
with creamed nut icing flavoured with
mixed spice, and walnuts. No spice is
needed if you are making a coconut icing.

CREAMED COCONUT CAKE TOPPING

4 oz (115g) creamed coconut
2 tablespoons sunflower oil

1. Grate the coconut and blend in with
sunflower oil. For a softer, buttery texture
use three tablespoons oil.

2. Coconut flour, if mixed with a small
amount of oil, makes good edible 'snow' to
sprinkle over cake tops.

FRUITARIAN CAKE

6 oz (170g) chopped dates
6 oz (115g) chopped apricots
2 oz (55g) milled cashews
1 oz (30g) sunflower seeds or chopped
nuts (any kind)
Millet flakes or desiccated coconut

1. A strong pastry blender is the best to
use for this. Blend fruit, nuts and seeds
thoroughly and pound with heavy
wooden spoon or potato masher.

2. Flatten and roll in millet flakes or
desiccated coconut.

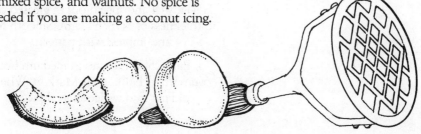

Banana Oatmeal Lunch Cake

The oatmeal makes the texture of this cake similar to that of Parkin.

1 level teaspoon cream of tartar
1 level teaspoon bicarbonate of soda
½ lb (225g) wholemeal flour
4 oz (115g) medium oatmeal
4 oz (115g) raw cane sugar
2 tablespoons treacle or syrup
4 oz (115g) dried bananas cut into thin rings
2 oz (55g) chopped peel
6 fl oz (170ml) oil
Approx 6 fl oz (170ml) cold water

1. Add cream of tartar and bicarbonate of soda to flour and add everything else except oil.

2. Pour in oil simultaneously with a similar volume of cold water and mix well. Add more water as necessary to make an easily beatable mixture. Beat well.

3. Bake in shallow baking tin lined with greaseproof paper for 45 minutes in oven at 400°F/200°C (Gas Mark 6).

Bruke Cake

½ lb (225g) wholemeal flour
4 oz (115g) medium oatmeal
4 oz (115g) raw cane sugar
Slightly less than 1 level teaspoon bicarbonate of soda
Slightly more than 1 level teaspoon cream of tartar
1 oz white fat
4 oz (115g) coconut flour
6 oz (170g) currants

1. Mix together dry ingredients, aerating and breaking up any lumps. Rub in fat.

2. Add coconut flour and washed currants.

3. Mix with cold water and beat well. Bake in flat oven tin 45 minutes at 400°F/200°C (Gas Mark 6).

Maize Shortbread

4 oz (115g) maizemeal
4 oz (115g) wholemeal flour
4 oz (115g) white fat
2 tablespoons syrup

1. Rub fat into maizemeal and wholemeal flour. Add syrup, then sufficient water to make soft dough.

2. Mix well and spread out in greased tin to thickness of ¾ inch (2cm). Smooth top and impress with pattern.

3. Bake 25-30 minutes in medium hot oven 375°F/190°C (Gas Mark 5). When cold cut into wedge-shaped pieces.

Brownie Bobbles

2 oz (55g) vegetable fat
1 oz (30g) Barbados sugar
4 oz (115g) milled cashews
4 oz (115g) soya flour
1 rounded teaspoon powdered coriander
2 tablespoons syrup
2 oz (55g) dates, chopped

1. Cream fat and sugar and blend with nuts, soya flour, coriander and syrup.

2. Form into small balls about ¾ inch (2cm) in diameter with a piece of date enclosed in each.

3. Cook slowly for 20-30 minutes at 300-325°F/150-170°C (Gas Mark 2-3) being careful they do not scorch. When cool put in an airtight tin and use within a week.

Chocolate Biscuits

4 oz white fat
4 oz (115g) wholemeal flour
4 oz (115g) oats
4 oz (115g) raw cane sugar
2 teaspoons baking powder
1 tablespoon cocoa

1. Rub fat into dry ingredients. Bind with water. Roll out. Cut into circles.

2. Bake at 400°F/200°C (Gas Mark 6), for about 12 minutes. The biscuits can have a little melted chocolate poured over when cold, if desired.

Spice Biscuits

4 oz (115g) wholemeal flour
4 oz (115g) oats
4 oz (115g) raw cane sugar
1 teaspoon mixed spice
¾ teaspoon bicarbonate of soda
1 level teaspoon cream of tartar
4 oz vegetable suet
1 small tablespoon black treacle

1. Mix dry ingredients. Stir in suet. Dissolve treacle in a little cold water and mix in.

2. Roll out ¼ inch (5mm) thick and cut into rounds 2¼ inch (5.5cm) diameter. Bake on greased sheet 10-15 minutes at 375°F/190°C (Gas Mark 5) being careful not to burn. Allow to cool slightly before removing to wire cooling tray. Store in airtight tin.

USEFUL INFORMATION

THE VEGAN SOCIETY
(FOUNDED 1944)

Advocates living on the products of the plant kingdom to the exclusion of all food and other commodities derived wholly or in part from animals. Its members base their lives on the ethic of Reverence for Life and seek to free themselves from all forms of cruelty and exploitation. They are aware of man's responsibilities to his environment and seek to promote the proper use of the resources of the earth.

The Vegan Society was formed in 1944 and has a world-wide membership which is now growing more rapidly than ever before. Through its Council, staff, local contacts and publications it helps members to practise a healthy way of life, to find fellowship with each other and to spread its message which is being more and more recognized as urgent and vital if man is to meet the challenge of the environmental crisis.

Free information (stamp appreciated) is available from:

The Secretary
The Vegan Society
7 Battle Road
St Leonards-on-Sea
East Sussex
TN37 7AA

British and American Equivalents

This book was written for a British readership. To help the American cook with the system of measurement used, the following conversion table shows American cup equivalents for liquid measures.

British	American
8 fl oz	1 cup
1/2 pint/10 fl oz	1 1/4 cups
16 fl oz	1 pint
1 pint/20 fl oz	2 1/2 cups
2 pints/40 fl oz	5 cups
8 tablespoons	1/2 cup

INDEX

143